Good Cholesterol,
Bad Cholesterol

Also by Anita Hirsch

Drink to Your Health

Other books in the "Good, Bad" series

Good Fats, Bad Fats by Rosemary Stanton, Ph.D.

Good Carbs, Bad Carbs by Johanna Burani, M.S., R.D.,
C.D.E and Linda Rao, M.Ed.

Good Stress, Bad Stress by Barry Lenson

Anita Hirsch, M.S., R.D.

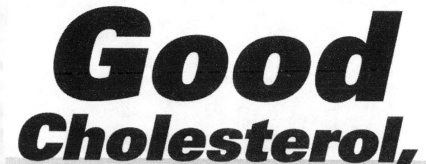

Good
Cholesterol,

An Indispensable
Guide to the Facts about
Cholesterol

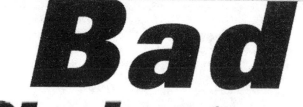

Bad
Cholesterol

MARLOWE & COMPANY
NEW YORK

Published by
Marlowe & Company
An Imprint of Avalon Publishing Group Incorporated
161 William Street, 16th Floor
New York, NY 10038

Library of Congress Cataloging-in-Publication Data
Hirsch, Anita, M.S.
Good cholesterol, bad cholesterol / Anita Hirsch.
p. cm.
Includes index.
ISBN 1-56924-528-2 (trade paper)
1. Hypercholesteremia—Popular works. 2. Blood cholesterol—
Popular works. I. Title.
RC632.H83 H55 2002
616.3'997—dc21   2002020112

Designed by Pauline Neuwirth, Neuwirth & Associates, Inc.

Printed in the United States of America

CONTENTS

INTRODUCTION

At some point in your life, you will probably take a serious interest in cholesterol. During a routine physical exam, the customary blood test may reveal an abnormal cholesterol number. Usually the word *cholesterol* is paired with *high* and then *avoid heart disease,* and a prescription for a cholesterol-lowering drug follows.

But this scenario is not inevitable. If you modify your lifestyle now, you may be able to avoid ever hearing the words *high cholesterol,* and ever having to take cholesterol-lowering drugs—as well as reduce your risks for heart disease.

America's number-one killer is cardiovascular disease, which includes high blood pressure, coronary heart disease (heart attack and angina), stroke, congenital heart defects, and congestive heart failure. One in four Americans has some form of cardiovascular disease, accounting for more than 40 percent of all deaths each year in the United States. Most of our health care dollars are going toward fighting cardiovascular disease.

The American Heart Association advises Americans to quit smoking, use beta blockers after a heart attack, control high blood pressure, and keep track of and control cholesterol if coronary heart disease is present. If you keep your cholesterol level in the desirable range, maintain a healthy weight, exercise, and avoid smoking, you can lessen your chances for succumbing to heart disease.

Good Cholesterol, Bad Cholesterol is aimed at those who want to understand cholesterol better, who desire to keep their cholesterol low, who are committed to good health, and who hope to extend their lives.

The book is divided into two parts. The first is an explanation of cholesterol that includes the various forms of cholesterol and the definition of terms. The second part is the practical part, or what *you* can do about cholesterol. You can check out your risk of heart disease in the next ten years. Or you can look in the Appendix for a list of foods with their cholesterol, fat, saturated fat, omega fat, and trans fat content.

This book will try to iron out all the questions you may have about cholesterol: the good and the bad. Your total cholesterol level is not the only thing your physician is interested in. The doctor may also talk about HDL, or the "good" cholesterol—and next, the LDL, or the "bad" cholesterol. What are those numbers? And what do they mean?

I hope that by the time you are finished reading this book, you will understand cholesterol and have answers to all your questions about it. I also hope you will soon attain desirable cholesterol and LDL numbers. If I can help you achieve this goal, my own goal in writing this book will have been achieved.

ANITA HIRSCH M.S., R.D.
April 2002

PART 1:

What's Cholesterol, Anyway?

FATS AND YOUR HEALTH

What Is Cholesterol and How Does It Affect Health?

Cholesterol, LDL, HDL, *triglycerides, omega-3, polyunsaturated fatty acids.* You've read about them in the newspaper. You've heard about them on TV. This one is good and that one is bad. Or is it the other way around? What do all these things really mean, anyway? Can anyone who isn't a research scientist with an MD and a couple of Ph.D. degrees really understand all this stuff?

Sure they can. Once you understand the basics, all the other terms seem to fall into place. So let's get started with the main topic of this book: cholesterol.

Cholesterol is a waxy, fat-like substance that belongs to a family of chemicals called **lipids**, which do not mix with water. Lipids, including cholesterol, are found in every part of your body. As I explain later, you need cholesterol to live. However, sometimes you can have too much of a good thing. High levels of cholesterol in the blood are dangerous, because this fatty substance can build up in your blood vessels—the arteries and veins—which carry oxygen and nutrients to every cell in your body. An accumulation of cholesterol and other substances, called **plaque**, makes the vessels narrower and narrower, reducing the flow of blood. It may eventually block the vessels completely.

A **heart attack** occurs when there is a blockage of blood to the heart.

A **stroke** occurs when there is a blockage of blood to the brain.

How Does a Blockage Happen in the Veins and Arteries?

When you are young, the insides of your arteries are smooth, and the blood can move freely through them. Over a period of years, cholesterol, fat, calcium, and other substances in the blood may be deposited in the inner walls of the arteries that supply blood to the heart and to the brain. Once these deposits begin and a rough surface is formed, the blood may coagulate around it and form a clot. As the clot enlarges, it limits or eventually shuts off the blood supply. A clot can break loose, and when it moves through a narrowed artery it cuts off the blood supply completely.

Coronary heart disease or a heart attack occurs when one or more of the blood vessels in the heart, the **coronary arteries**, partially or completely close. Oxygen and nutrients cannot reach the parts of the heart where the blockages are, and some of the heart muscle may die. As a result, the heart becomes weaker and cannot pump nutrient-rich blood out to the body.

You do not know that the arteries are building up plaque: you may not have any symptoms. More than two-thirds of the arteries might be clogged before you would feel any distress. Stress or physical exertion may cause pain or pressure, referred to as **angina,** when the blood going through the arteries in the heart is slowed down and the heart muscle can't get as much oxygen as it needs.

About Atherosclerosis

With age, arteries may become hardened and thickened. This is **artherosclerosis,** or **arteriosclerosis,** popularly called *hard-*

ening of the arteries. The word sclerosis just means "hardening." The word *arteriosclerosis* says nothing about the cause of the hardening.

When lipids gather along the inner walls of the arteries and form plaques that make the walls of the arteries lose their elasticity and harden, the result is atherosclerosis (the formal name for plaque is *atheroma*). If the process is unchecked, coronary heart disease results.

Normally, as blood pulses through the arteries, they expand as the pressure increases. But when arteries harden, they can't expand, and the blood pressure rises. The increase in blood pressure is a strain on the heart.

Sometimes as the pressure builds, a part of an artery can balloon out where it has been weakened. This is referred to as an **aneurysm**. An aneurysm can burst and lead to internal bleeding and death.

Front View of Heart Showing Cross Sections of Arteries

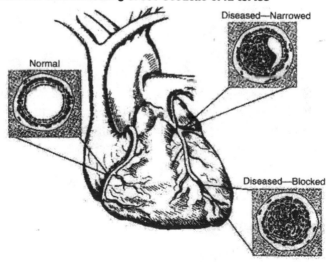

Source: The National Institutes of Health, NHLBI

Our Bodies Do Need Cholesterol

Although high levels of blood cholesterol are dangerous, you do need some cholesterol. Cholesterol is responsible for the production of the hormones testosterone and estrogen, vitamin D, and bile acids. Bile acids are substances produced in the liver and used in the intestine to help digest fat.

Your body manufactures cholesterol in the liver. The more cholesterol you eat, the less cholesterol your body produces. The less cholesterol you eat, the more the body produces.

Your body is smart, even when your eating habits are not. Even if you stop eating cholesterol, if you continue to eat a lot of saturated fat (described later), your body produces cholesterol. If you continue to eat more saturated fat than your body needs and you do not exercise to burn it off, you just get heavier and fatter because the extra fat is deposited in your fat cells and stored there until you need it.

Keep Cholesterol out of the Blood

Most Americans get their dietary cholesterol from whole or low-fat milk, whole or low-fat dairy products (cheeses, sour cream, yogurt), eggs, butter, beef, poultry, fish, and deli meats. The cholesterol in foods and the cholesterol that is produced by your liver raise blood levels of cholesterol. It is the cholesterol that appears in your blood, referred to as **serum cholesterol** or **blood cholesterol** (the terms mean essentially the same thing), that is the cholesterol you want to avoid.

The First Steps for Preventing High Blood Cholesterol

- Cut out smoking
- Keep your weight down
- Exercise

You will notice that the first three steps to avoiding high blood cholesterol are not concerned with eating cholesterol or particular fats. It is overeating in general that leads to the weight gain that gets people into trouble, especially if they are eating high amounts of fat, high amounts of saturated fat, and too many calories.

To prevent weight gain and to lower blood cholesterol you need to change the kinds of foods you eat. Cutting down on the consumption of high-cholesterol foods and high-fat foods can be the first step to avoid or lower high blood cholesterol. The key is to eat the right type of fat and also to eat less fat or only enough to keep you healthy. Changing your diet is covered in more detail in Chapters 8, 9, and 10.

Where to Find Cholesterol

Cholesterol is found *only* in animal products. The following table shows some sources of cholesterol. The egg is high in cholesterol but low in fat. Beef is lower in cholesterol but has more fat, and of the 30 grams of fat in the high-fat prime rib, almost half, about 13 grams, is saturated fat.

High-cholesterol shrimp is very low in fat, and less than 1 gram is saturated fat. Choose foods that are the lowest in cholesterol as well as lowest in saturated fat.

The National Heart, Lung and Blood Institute recommends that the daily intake of cholesterol for adults should be 300 mg or less per day. In their latest set of recommendations (from 2002), part of the National Cholesterol Education Program, they add that if you already have high blood cholesterol, the recommended intake of cholesterol is 200 mg per day. Look over the foods in the table and see which ones can fit into your diet.

You will also want to keep your intake of fat low, particularly if you are overweight. A food that has 3 grams of fat or less per serving is considered "low fat."

The Cholesterol, Fat, and Saturated Fat in Certain Foods

Food	Amount	Cholesterol (mg)	Fat (g)	Saturated Fat (g)
Liver	3 oz.	331	4	2
Egg	1	212	5	2
Shrimp	3 oz.	165	1	0.2
Veal	3 oz.	100	15	8
Prime rib	3 oz.	72	30	13
Chicken (no skin)	3 oz.	72	3	1
Sausage	3 oz.	71	27	9
Fish (baked haddock)	3 oz.	60	1	0.1
Ice cream	1 cup	58	15	9
Milk (whole)	1 cup	33	8	5
Hamburger (lean)	3 oz.	31	8	5
Butter	1 tbs.	31	12	7
Cheese (cheddar)	1 oz.	30	9	6
Milk (2 percent)	1 cup	18	5	3
Cake doughnut	1	17	11	2
Milk (1 percent)	1 cup	10	3	2
Blue cheese dressing	2 tbs.	5	16	3
Milk (skim)	1 cup	4	0.4	0.3
Soft light margarine	1 tbs.	0	4.5	0
Regular margarine	1 tbs.	0	11	2
Chunky peanut butter	2 tbs.	0	16	4

Source: ESHA and food labels

What Is a Saturated Fat?

I've already mentioned that you should avoid **saturated fat**. To understand what saturated fat is, you first have to understand what fat is. The basic units of fats and oils are called **fatty acids.** Each type of fat or oil has a combination of saturated or unsaturated fatty acids in it. Usually three fatty acids are connected together to make a fat, which is also referred to as a **triglyceride**. Throughout this book I will use the terms *fats, fatty acids,* and *triglycerides* interchangeably because from a nutritional point of view they are approximately the same.

Saturated fatty acids are found in higher amounts in animal products such as meat, poultry, milk, lard, and butter, but saturated fats *are* found in vegetable products. The vegetable oils in coconut, palm kernel, and palm oils consist mainly of saturated fats. Saturated fats are usually solid at room temperature, and these are the fats to avoid because they raise the serum cholesterol and bad cholesterol (LDL) the most.

Notice in the table above that there are different amounts of saturated fats in the high- and low-fat foods. The low-fat egg contains 2 grams of saturated fat and so does the high-fat doughnut.

The table below shows the amounts of saturated fat in different oils.

Where the Saturated Fat Is

Fat	Percent Saturated
Canola oil	sss 7%
Safflower oil	sssss 9%
Flaxseed oil	sssss 10%
Sunflower	ssssss 12%
Corn oil	sssssss 14%
Olive oil	sssssss 14%
Soybean	sssssss 14%
Margarine (soft)	sssssss 14%
Margarine (hard)	ssssssss 16%
Peanut oil	sssssssss 19%
Crisco (can)	ssssssssssss 25%
Cottonseed oil	sssssssssssss 26%
Chicken fat	sssssssssssss 30%

Fat	Percent Saturated
Lard	sssssssssssssssssssss 40%
Palm oil	ssssssssssssssssssssssss 50%
Beef fat	ssssssssssssssssssssssss 51%
Butter	ssssssssssssssssssssssss 51%
Chocolate	sssssssssssssssssssssssssss 60 %
Coconut oil	ssssssssssssssssssssssssssssssssssssssssss 88%

Source: ESHA Research, Inc.

What Is the Difference between Saturated and Unsaturated Fats?

Now let's look a little closer at the chemistry of the fats. Fats are combinations of carbon, hydrogen, and oxygen. In the fatty acids that make up fats, carbon atoms are linked together like a chain. Chemists call these links *bonds.* When the chain contains as many hydrogens as possible, chemists call the fats *saturated.* It means the chain is saturated with hydrogen.

If it is possible to attach more hydrogens to the chain, that means the chain is not saturated with hydrogen, these fats are called **unsaturated fats.**

What Is a Monounsaturated Fat?

If an unsaturated fat has only one place where more hydrogen can attach, it is referred to as a **monounsaturated fat**. If it has two or more places where hydrogens can attach, it is called a **polyunsaturated fat**.

All the vegetable oils contain a combination of unsaturated (polyunsaturated and monounsaturated) fat and saturated fat. The more saturated fat that the oils contain, the firmer they are at room temperature.

The table below shows the amount of monounsaturated fats in different oils. Choose fats and oils that are highest in monounsaturated fats because they help lower cholesterol in the blood.

The oils that are highest in monounsaturated fatty acids are olive, canola, and peanut, in that order. The foods that are highest in monounsaturated fatty acids are avocados and nuts such as almonds, pecans, cashews, and peanuts.

Actually, beef fat is almost as high in monounsaturated fatty acids as peanut oil, but the other predominant fatty acid in beef is saturated, while the other fatty acid in peanut oil is mainly polyunsaturated. Because of the high saturated fat content of beef and because it is also high in fat in general, it should be limited or even omitted from the diet. It is what you do every day that counts. If you eat a beef hamburger every day for lunch, you should change your eating habits. A beef hamburger once a week is definitely the limit; and even once a month would be a healthier limit.

To lower blood cholesterol, choose an oil or fat that is lowest in saturated fat and highest in monounsaturated fat.

The following is a list of fats and oils with their monounsaturated fat content. Olive oil is the preferred oil since it is so high in monounsaturated fat. Remember, all fats are a combination of saturated and unsaturated fats.

Where the Monounsaturated Fat Is

Fat	Percent Saturated
Olive oil	MMMMMMMMMMMMMMMMMMMMMMMMMMMMM 74%
Canola oil	MMMMMMMMMMMMMMMMMMMMMMMMMMMMMM 59%
Peanut oil	MMMMMMMMMMMMMMMMMMMMMMMM 46%
Chicken fat	MMMMMMMMMMMMMMMMMMMMMMM 45%
Crisco (can)	MMMMMMMMMMMMMMMMMMMMMMM 45%
Beef fat	MMMMMMMMMMMMMMMMMMMMMM 43%
Lard	MMMMMMMMMMMMMMMMMMMM 42%
Palm oil	MMMMMMMMMMMMMMMMMM 39%
Margarine (hard)	MMMMMMMMMMMMMMMMM 36%

Fat	Percent Saturated
Chocolate	MMMMMMMMMMMMMMMMMM 30%
Margarine (soft)	MMMMMMMMMMMMMMMMM 29%
Corn oil	MMMMMMMMMMMMMM 25%
Butter	MMMMMMMMMMMMM 24%
Soybean oil	MMMMMMMMMMMM 23%
Sunflower oil	MMMMMMMMMM 20%
Cottonseed oil	MMMMMMMMMM 20%
Flaxseed oil	MMMMMMMMM 17%
Safflower oil	MMMMMM 12%
Chocolate	MMMMM 10%
Coconut oil	MMM 6%

Source: ESHA Research, Inc.

What Is a Polyunsaturated Fat?

As described earlier, polyunsaturated fats are unsaturated fats with two or more bonds where hydrogen can be added. Polyunsaturated fats are usually liquid at room temperature. Two of the polyunsaturated fatty acids, **linoleic** (omega-6; the omega fatty acids are described in the following sections) and **alpha-linolenic** (omega-3), are necessary for making hormones and cells. These two fatty acids are called **essential fatty acids** because your body is unable to make them, so they must be eaten in foods.

Oils, such as flaxseed, safflower, sunflower, and corn, are high in polyunsaturated fatty acids, including the essential fatty acids. Foods that contain these essential fatty acids are eggs, fish, fruit, vegetables, and grains.

The polyunsaturated fats you buy in the store, such as corn oil, safflower oil, flaxseed oil, and sunflower oil, are referred to as **refined vegetable oils**. The refined oils get rancid easily and must be treated with care. This means refrigerating them and not storing them for a long time. Commercial vegetable oils are often deodorized to remove the smell of rancidity, according to lipid researcher Mary G. Enig, Ph.D.

Vegetable oils are used widely as cooking oils and in salad dressing, baked goods, and snack foods, so scientists think that Americans are eating enough polyunsaturated oils in their diets to satisfy the requirement for essential fatty acids.

Just one tablespoon of polyunsaturated vegetable oil in a salad, margarine, or other foods in a normal diet satisfies an adult's daily requirement for linoleic acid (omega-6), the major essential fatty acid.

What Are Omega-3 Fatty Acids?

There are two major types of polyunsaturated fats: the omega-3 and the omega-6 types.

The omega-3s are found in soy oil, canola oil, flaxseed oil, or in fish, a particularly good source being fatty ocean fish such as salmon, sardines, mackerel, herring, and albacore tuna. The omega-3s are the ones that reduce the risk of dying from a heart attack. They are known to benefit heart health by reducing blood fats and making the blood less likely to clot.

You need to eat two servings, or about 7 ounces, of the fatty ocean fish a week to help prevent blood clots. Because fish also contain saturated fat and cholesterol, you do not want to go overboard with fatty fish consumption either. More is not better.

Fish oil supplements also can supply the omega-3 fatty acids, but it is best to get the essential fatty acids from foods. Omega-3 fatty acids are also found in nuts and green leafy vegetables.

Where the Omega-3 Fatty Acids Are

Food	Amount	Omega-3 Fatty Acid (g)
English walnuts	¼ cup	2.72
Atlantic mackerel (baked)	3 oz.	1.12
Salmon (canned, drained)	3 oz.	1.06
Farmed rainbow trout	3 oz.	1.05
Tuna (white, canned, drained)	3 oz.	.84
Blue mussels	3 oz.	.39
Atlantic halibut Filet (raw)	3 oz.	.36
Atlantic sardines (*in oil, drained*)	2	.36
Shrimp (steamed)	3 oz.	.36
Pecans	¼ cup	.20
Atlantic cod (baked)	3 oz.	.14
Cantaloupe (cubed)	1 cup	.10
Kale (boiled)	½ cup	.07
Spinach (boiled)	½ cup	.05
Broccoli (chopped raw)	½ cup	.05

Source: ESHA Research, Inc.

What Are Omega-6 Fatty Acids?

The other essential polyunsaturated fatty acids are the omega-6 fatty acids, which help lower blood cholesterol levels. The omega-6s are found in corn, sunflower, and safflower oils. They are also found in many foods including eggs, fish, fruits, vegetables, legumes, and grains. In fact, the omega-6 fatty acids are in so many foods—especially in prepared supermarket and restaurant foods—that no one needs to worry about not getting enough of these essential fatty acids.

The ratio of the omega-3 and the omega-6 fatty acids that you eat is important. People who eat less of the omega-6 fats—found in the corn and sunflower oil used in packaged foods—and more of the omega-3 fatty acids—healthful fats found in foods such as fatty fish, walnuts, flaxseed oil, and green leafy vegetables—are actually at reduced risk for heart disease and macular degeneration.

Hence, *don't overdo your consumption of omega-6 fats*. That means read the labels on foods and if they are high in fat—unless the fats are only the healthier oils such as olive or canola oils—then it would be best to avoid them. In Japan, people have been known for their long lives. However, their traditional diet of rice and fish has been changing. Now more prosperous, they are adding vegetable oils and processed foods to their diet, which brings more omega-6 fatty acids into their diet. Researchers in Japan are blaming an increase in heart disease and other problems such as cancer, asthma, and allergies on the increase of omega-6 oils in the diet.

The Major Types of Polyunsaturated Fats, Their Sources, and Their Impact on Health

Polyunsaturated Fats			
Omega-6	**Omega-3**		
	alpha-linolenic acid (ALA)	eicosapentaenoic acid (EPA)	docosahexaenoic acid (DHA)
↓	↓	↓	↓
Corn oil Safflower oil Sunflower oil	Flaxseed oil Soybean oil Canola oil	Salmon, Sardines, Mackerel, Herring, Albacore Tuna	
↓	↓	↓	↓
Help lower serum cholesterol; Americans get plenty of these	Reduce risk of dying from heart disease; most Americans need to eat more of these.		

Source: Communicating Food for Health Newsletter copyright www.foodandhealth.com

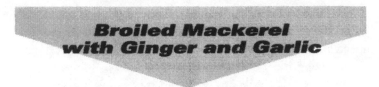

Broiled Mackerel with Ginger and Garlic

This recipe is high in omega-3 fatty acids.

THERE ARE SEVERAL kinds of mackerel, all coming from the Atlantic Ocean. The one referred to as Atlantic mackerel has a strong flavor and more of the omega-3 fatty acids than other varieties. It lives in waters off the northeastern United States. The wahoo, cero, and Spanish mackerel are white and have a mild flavor when cooked. They live in waters around Florida. The Boston and Spanish varieties are more easily found in local markets. The wahoo is a larger fish, like the tuna, and is found in the warmer waters; in Hawaii the wahoo is known as ono.

Mackerel are fattest in the fall; over the winter they lose their fat, so by spring they are lean. In other words, the mackerel probably contain the most omega-3 fatty acids in the fall.

It is best to buy fish fresh, from a reliable retailer, and use it within two days. If you have to freeze fish, wrap it well in a heavy plastic bag or moisture-proof wrapping and use it within four months.

Note that King Mackerel, the large and more mature fish, is the mackerel variety that is high in mercury and should be avoided by pregnant women, nursing mothers, women who may become pregnant, and young children.

1 lb.	Spanish mackerel fillets
2 tbs.	lemon juice
2 tsp.	light soy sauce
2 cloves	garlic, minced
2 tsp.	grated fresh ginger
	Lemon wheels, garnish

1. Rinse the Spanish mackerel fillets, remove the skin, and cut into 4 portions. Place them on the broiler pan.
2. Combine the lemon juice, soy sauce, garlic, and ginger. Spoon over the fish.
3. Broil the fish for 4 minutes about 4 to 5 inches from the heat. Then turn carefully. Spoon any remaining marinade over the fish and broil for 4 to 5 more minutes or until the fish is cooked through.
4. Serve garnished with thinly sliced lemon.

{ Yield: 4 servings }

Per serving: 164 calories, 2 g carbohydrate, 7 g fat, 2 g sat fat, 3 g poly fat, 3 g mono fat, 86 mg cholesterol, 0 dietary fiber, 156 mg sodium, 2 g omega-3 fatty acids.

What Is a Trans Fatty Acid?

Vegetable oils that are liquid at room temperature can be changed into solid fats by adding hydrogen. This is how vegetable oil is converted into vegetable shortening or margarine. Chemists say that the links have been **hydrogenated.** When not all the links have been hydrogenated, the products are **partially hydrogenated.** Some of these partially hydrogenated products contain fats called **trans fats.**

On nutrition labels, you'll often see *partially hydrogenated vegetable oils* included in the ingredient list. Margarine, crackers, and cookies all contain partially hydrogenated vegetable shortening.

How Bad Are the Trans Fats?

Trans fatty acids are thought to be as harmful as saturated fatty acids. They can be used to make cholesterol and are related to the development of heart disease.

Dietary Sources of Trans Fat

According to the American Heart Association, the four most commonly eaten foods that are the source of trans fatty acids in the diet are:

1. Margarine
2. Beef, pork, lamb as a main dish
3. Cookies (biscuits)
4. White bread

Food labels are not required to include the amount of trans fatty acids on them. If you want to know how much trans fat is in a commercial product such as a cracker, cookie, or margarine, you can estimate it from the Nutrition Facts label. For example, in the table below, there are 5 grams of fat in a serving of 15 crackers. By adding the saturated (1 g), polyunsaturated (0 g), and monounsaturated (1.5 g) fats on the label you get a total fat of 2.5 grams. Subtracting that total from the total fat listed on the label, which is 5 grams, you get a remainder of 2.5 grams. This 2.5 grams is the trans fat. In other words, half of the fat in the crackers is trans fat. Although these crackers are low in fat in general, you will want to watch that you don't eat too many.

Calculating Trans Fat from a Nutrition Facts Label

(The amounts are for 15 crackers or a serving)

Total fat from label	5
From label (sat, poly, mono)	-2.5 g
(1 g) (0 g) (1.5 g)	
Total trans fat	2.5 g

Restaurant foods and fast foods do not have nutritional labels on them and could contain high levels of trans fatty acids. For example:

One doughnut	3.2 g trans fatty acids
Large fries	6.8 g trans fatty acids
TOTAL	10.0 g trans fatty acids

How to Cut Down on the Amount of Trans Fatty Acids You Eat

The American Heart Association suggests the following steps for cutting down on your trans fatty acid consumption:

1. Use naturally occurring, unhydrogenated oils as much as possible: olive, canola, peanut, etc.
2. Look for processed foods made with oil. Avoid hydrogenated or saturated fats such as lard, coconut oil, palm oil, and palm kernel oil.
3. Use margarine instead of butter and choose soft (tub or liquid) margarine with no more than 2 grams of saturated fat per tablespoon, and with liquid oil as the first ingredient.
4. Avoid French fries, doughnuts, cookies, crackers, and baked goods that are commercially made.
5. Limit the fat in your diet.
6. Avoid fast food, since commercially used shortenings and deep frying fats are hydrogenated and contain trans fat.

If you follow these six rules you will lower your trans fat intake and also limit your intake of fat and saturated fat—and lower your blood cholesterol, too.

THE GOOD AND THE BAD: HDL, LDL, AND VLDL

Cholesterol is a fatty substance, so it cannot dissolve in water, or in blood. Hence cholesterol travels in your blood through the arteries and veins in units called **lipoproteins**, which are a combination of fat and protein. There are three major types of lipoprotein: **high-density lipoprotein (HDL),** often called "good cholesterol," **low-density lipoprotein (LDL),** called "bad cholesterol," and **very low density lipoprotein (VLDL).**

High-Density Lipoproteins

HDLs are the *"good"* cholesterol because HDL cholesterol helps transport cholesterol, particularly the LDL or "bad" cholesterol, out of the blood and back to the liver, where it is removed from the body or reprocessed. The liver processes the LDL into other compounds that the body needs to function. In other words, HDL prevents cholesterol from building up in the arteries. HDL even removes excess cholesterol from artery walls, so I call it the Heart's De-Lite.

One point of interest here is that fat in the diet stimulates the production of HDL. If you lower your fat intake too much, your HDL will go down. Some researchers suggest substituting a better fat—an oil high in monounsaturated fat such as olive oil—for stick margarine and the other fats and oils in your diet. They say that if you add more olive oil, or increase your fat intake to 30 to 35 percent of the calories from fat, your HDL will go up.

The problem with adding fat to your diet is that it is difficult to know when you have achieved 30 to 35 percent of your calories from fat. Since more than half of Americans are obese, I would not want to suggest eating more fat, which translates to more calories, but I would suggest substituting a better fat.

Other than smoking and a sedentary lifestyle, the third major risk factor for high cholesterol is weighing too much. So if you are overweight, one of your goals should be to lose weight.

A low-fat diet (for examples of menus with a low fat content, see Chapter 10) can help with weight loss because there are more calories in fat than in protein and carbohydrate. If you are eating less fat and also using some low-fat or fat-free products, you should be losing weight, especially if you are not eating more food to make up for the lower calorie level. Often, while you are losing weight your LDL cholesterol will go down, and so will your HDL. When your weight has stabilized, your HDL should rise.

Another reason for low HDL may be that you are genetically predisposed to low HDL. Your doctor can help you if heredity is the problem.

What Is the Best HDL Score?

It is best if your blood HDL cholesterol is higher than 40 mg/dL (mg/dL stands for "milligrams per deciliter"). An HDL level under 40 mg/dL increases your heart disease risk. And if the "Hearts De-Lite" cholesterol is higher than 60 mg/dL, you have one less risk factor for heart disease and have lowered your chance of getting heart disease. Keep up whatever you are doing!

Low-Density Lipoproteins

LDL is referred to as the *"bad"* cholesterol, because too much LDL in the blood can injure blood vessel walls and can lead to cholesterol buildup and blockage of the arteries. LDLs, or as I like to call these lipoproteins, the "Low Down Lousy" type, carry most of the cholesterol in the blood. Modifying your diet is the best way to achieve a lower LDL and a healthier you. I describe modifying your diet in Chapters 8, 9, and 10.

New studies show that the LDL units traveling in the blood are a major cause of coronary heart disease, and deaths from heart disease can be cut if the "bad" cholesterol is lowered with aggressive treatment. So if you want to avoid a heart attack, you should lower your LDL levels.

What Is the Best LDL Number?

The best blood LDL level for men and women is 100 mg/dL or lower. Studies have shown that women with elevated LDL levels in the blood are more liable to have heart disease than men with the same high levels. After men and women reach seventy-five years, a higher cholesterol level is protective and is related to lower mortality.

Very Low Density Lipoprotein

VLDL is the lipoprotein package that transports **triglycerides** (the scientific name for fats) from the liver through the blood to the organs that need them. High levels of triglycerides have been linked to increased risk of heart disease. When the VLDL leaves the liver, it is loaded with fat. Once the VLDL has dropped off the triglycerides at various cells (for example, muscle cells can burn triglycerides for energy, and fat cells store triglycerides for future use), the VLDL breaks down to LDL. These breakdown particles can cling to the artery walls and cause the clogging of the arteries called atherosclerosis (described earlier).

What Is the Best VLDL Score?

The VLDL score on your blood test is part of the triglyceride number, which should be lower than 150 mg/dL. Triglycerides are explained in the next chapter. Most labs currently do not report a VLDL score.

What Is the "Metabolic Syndrome" and Do You Have It?

The latest guidelines from the National Cholesterol Education Program state that if your HDL, or good cholesterol, scores are lower than forty, then you are at greater risk for heart disease and you may have what researchers are calling the "metabolic syndrome."

The Metabolic Syndrome

You have the syndrome and are more at risk for heart disease if you have three of these five characteristics:

- ➤ high triglycerides
- ➤ high blood pressure
- ➤ high blood sugar
- ➤ abdominal obesity
- ➤ low HDL score

How Important Are the Good and the Bad?

Beginning at age twenty, you should have your blood checked for your good cholesterol (HDL), bad cholesterol (LDL), and triglyceride (used to calculate VLDL) scores. According to the latest figures by the American Heart Association, cholesterol screening increased from 67.3 percent in 1991 to 70.8 percent in 1999. During the years when more people were screened, the stroke death rate fell 13 percent.

The studies attribute this fall in the stroke death rate to the fact that patients and especially doctors are paying more attention to the results of cholesterol screenings; and as more people are screened, the stroke death rate will go down even more.

Dr. Norman Sarachek, an excellent, recently retired cardiologist, said that if a patient's LDL was higher than 100 and the total cholesterol was over 200 *and* the person had a family history of heart disease, that was a wake-up call. His remedy was to immediately prescribe one of the statin drugs, which are used to lower cholesterol levels.

Can You Unclog Your Arteries?

You may wish to try to unclog your arteries or lower your cholesterol levels by lifestyle changes rather than starting with a drug. According to studies, clogged arteries can be prevented or even reversed by eating a diet that is:

- very low fat
- near-vegetarian
- high fiber

How to go about incorporating these three rules into your diet is explained in Chapters 8, 9, and 10.

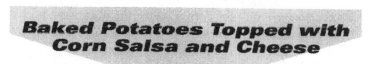

Baked Potatoes Topped with Corn Salsa and Cheese

A low-fat, near-vegetarian, high-fiber recipe

VEGETABLES ARE HIGH in dietary fiber, vitamins, minerals, and phytochemicals (see Chapter 8). One of the more popular *and* accepted vegetables eaten in the United States is the baked potato.

Potatoes are so popular that many people eat some form of them at every meal. Baking actually preserves more of the nutrients than most other methods of cooking do. Potatoes can be baked for an hour in the oven or they can be baked for 10 minutes in the microwave.

A variety of toppings make the baked potato a main dish. Scrambled egg substitute, chili, turkey barbecue, or a cheesy broccoli sauce are a few additions that "supreme" a potato. Instead of serving your entrees over rice, serve them on a baked potato. Even a thick soup, such as a lentil or chowder, will be a tasty addition to a baked potato.

2	large potatoes, baked
1	cup corn, frozen or canned
½ cup	chopped sweet red pepper
2 tbs.	chopped onion
2 tbs.	chopped tomato
2 tbs.	chopped fresh cilantro, optional
¼ tsp.	cumin
1 oz.	shredded low-fat cheddar cheese

1. After the potatoes are baked, cut them in half. Place them in a baking dish.
2. Combine the corn, sweet red pepper, chopped onion, chopped tomato, cilantro (if desired), and cumin. Top

the potatoes with the corn mixture. Finally, cover the corn mixture with the shredded cheese.

3. Place in the oven and bake for 10 minutes at 350°F until the cheese has melted and the corn mixture is hot.

❨ **Yield: 2 servings** ❩

Per serving: 344 calories, 12 g protein, 70 g carbohydrates, 8 g dietary fiber, 2 g soluble fiber, 8 g fat, 2 g saturated fat, 10 mg cholesterol, 306 mg sodium.

It is clearly in your best interest to pay attention to your LDL cholesterol and your HDL cholesterol scores and not just your total cholesterol level. If you have heart or artery disease in your family, you should use all possible means to lower your LDL.

Eat less, eat less fat, and eat less of the foods high in saturated fat. This should lower your LDL. Exercise and eliminate smoking. This should raise your HDL. Some people have high LDL scores because of their genes. Discuss your cholesterol scores with other family members. If others in your family have heart disease, talk to your doctor about your LDL.

3

TRIGLYCERIDES AND CHOLESTEROL

How do triglycerides fit into the picture? How do they help or hinder your good health? After you get the results of a blood test, look at the total cholesterol, the HDL, the LDL, and the triglyceride levels. High triglyceride levels—as well as high cholesterol levels—have been found to be a risk factor for coronary heart disease.

Triglycerides are the form in which most fats in food and in the body are found. Saturated, unsaturated, polyunsaturated, and monounsaturated fatty acids are all included in triglycerides. So when we talk about fat, we are really talking about triglycerides.

Recommended triglyceride level:

Less than 150 mg/dL

High Triglycerides Can Predict Heart Attack and Strokes

High blood triglyceride levels are a serious risk factor for heart disease. Even if your cholesterol level is normal, if your triglyceride level is high, you need to make some changes. Both cholesterol and triglycerides contribute to blood vessel clogging.

According to the American Heart Association, there is evidence that elevated blood triglyceride levels in a family can predict a heart attack-induced death years in advance.

Several new studies have shown that a high triglyceride level can also predict strokes. In a study led by David Tanne, M.D., involving more than 11,000 people with heart disease in Chaim Sheba Medical Center in Tel-Hashomer, Israel, researchers found that those with triglyceride levels over 200 were 30 percent more likely to have a stroke in the next 6 to 8 years. Those in whom the HDL level was over 40 mg/dL had fewer strokes.

How, If I Eat A Low-Fat Diet, Can I Still Have High Triglycerides?

Tryglycerides are a form of fat that the body makes from sugar and other carbohydrates, alcohol, or excess calories. So when you eat too much, even too many carbohydrates—too much sugar or too much bread, in other words, too many calories— the body can turn it into triglycerides (fat).

To make triglycerides or body fat, your body needs enzymes and a food source containing carbon, hydrogen, and oxygen. These three elements are the basis of all nutrients and organic matter. Sugar, which is also made of carbon, hydrogen, and oxygen, can be processed into fat by the body. In fact, some enzymes use any excess blood sugar to make fat.

The health problems that are related to high triglycerides include the metabolic syndrome, diabetes, high blood pressure, obesity, chronic kidney disease, and circulatory disease.

Bad Combinations: High Cholesterol and High Triglycerides Low HDL and High Triglycerides

Stephen Motsay, M.D., a family practice physician, says that "triglyceride levels we used to consider acceptable are now linked to a higher heart disease risk, especially if your cholesterol is high, too." Another bad combination and a heart disease risk is a low HDL level (below 40 mg/dL) and a high triglyceride level.

If your triglycerides are high, you probably have high total cholesterol as well as high LDL and low HDL. People with heart disease or diabetes or who are overweight usually already have a high triglyceride level. High triglyceride levels are more of a predictor of heart disease in women than in men, especially middle-aged women.

What Raises Blood Triglycerides?

The following will raise your blood trigylceride levels:

▶ a high-fat meal
▶ a high-calorie meal
▶ a high alcohol intake (for example, at a cocktail party)
▶ stress
▶ illness
▶ medication
▶ hormones
▶ menstrual cycle
▶ time of day
▶ recent exercise

If you have your blood tested during or after one of the items listed above—if, for example, you have blood drawn just after eating a high-fat meal or after a cocktail party, the triglyceride level may go through the roof.

When you eat a high-fat or high-calorie meal, the triglycerides move around in the blood for several hours afterward. If you already have plaque in your arteries, these triglycerides can easily attach to the walls of the vessels and increase your risk of a blockage or clot forming during that time.

Have You Eaten a High-Fat Meal Lately?

Many folks like to treat themselves to a special Sunday brunch or even a brunch buffet. Other than the coffee and juice, which have no fat, the items available might include prebuttered toast, bagels with cream cheese, omelettes, bacon, sausage, eggs Benedict, croissants, coffee cakes, and cheesecakes. A breakfast of these high-fat and high-calorie items would cause the blood triglycerides to rise for several hours.

According to Dr. Motsay, a complete lipid profile—total cholesterol, triglycerides, HDL, and LDL—should be checked in early adulthood. "If the results are normal, you need a retest about every three to five years. If your lipids are high, ask your doctor how often you should be tested. The decision is based on other risk factors such as smoking, hypertension, diabetes, family history of heart disease, obesity, and stress."

Another High-Fat Breakfast: Potato Chips

Lately I have noticed people eating potato chips for breakfast. They don't call it breakfast, but it is their first meal of the day: chips and soda.

On the way to work, they eat a bag of chips on the bus, or they stop for a refueling for the car and themselves: gasoline and a bag of chips at the local gas station.

Look at the Nutrition Facts on a 5-ounce bag of lightly salted gourmet chips, made with "expeller pressed high monounsaturated safflower and/or sunflower oil." The words may sound healthier, but they still are high in calories and fat.

The chip label says that 1 ounce (one serving) provides 150 calories, 9 grams of fat, and 110 mg of sodium. But who can eat just one—ounce, that is? I would say that it is difficult to stop at 5 ounces, which is the whole bag! 750 calories, 45 grams of fat, and 550 mg of sodium later you will still be hungry!

What Should You Do if Your Tryglycerides Are High?

> ➤ Lose excess weight (even 5 to 10 pounds will help)
> ➤ Exercise regularly
> ➤ Cut down on fats and sweets; focus on fiber
> ➤ Drink less alcohol
> ➤ If you have diabetes, get your blood sugar under control
> ➤ Eat one to two servings a week of fish rich in omega-3 fatty acids (salmon, mackerel, tuna, sardines)

Easy Salmon Salad

A quick, high omega-3, low-calorie recipe

7 oz. can	pink salmon with bones, no salt
½ cup	diced cucumber
3 tbs.	low-fat or nonfat mayonnaise
¼ cup	sliced green onion
2 cups	dark green lettuce
2 tomatoes	cut in wedges

Toss the salmon, cucumber, mayonnaise, and green onion together in a large mixing bowl. Refrigerate until ready to serve, up to 6 hours. Make a bed of lettuce and serve the salmon salad in the middle, garnished with tomatoes.

❨ **Yield: 2 servings** ❩

Per 1 cup serving: 187 calories, 8 g fat, 2 g sat fat, 23 mg cholesterol, 212 mg sodium, 11 g carbohydrate, 3 g fiber, 28 g protein, 1.8 g omega-3 fatty acids.

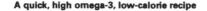

A high-fiber diet (see Chapter 9 for a table showing the fiber content of some common foods) will help to lower LDL and triglycerides. I can't reinforce that often enough. White flour, white bread, and white bagels—all low in fiber—are not helping you. Although whole wheat grains contain fiber, during processing to white flour, wheat loses fiber. Help yourself by eating plenty of foods with soluble fiber, such as beans, barley, oats, fruits, and vegetables.

There are two types of dietary fiber: soluble and insoluble. Soluble fiber is the type that lowers blood cholesterol and also delays sugar absorption. It is found mainly in fruits, vegetables, and legumes, especially in apples, oranges, and carrots. As I mentioned above, it is also found in oats and barley.

Insoluble fiber, which is good for keeping bowel movements regular and is good for the colon, doesn't dissolve in water, but it attracts water and speeds the elimination of waste products. The insoluble type helps prevent constipation and hemorrhoids. It is found in wheat bran and in the bran layer of most grains; in vegetable and fruit skins; and in whole grains, seeds, green peas, green beans, and nuts.

Foods can contain both types of fiber, and you need both. However, it is the soluble kind that is thought to lower cholesterol. Oat bran became popular several years ago because of its soluble fiber content.

Another way to help lower your triglyceride levels is to cut down on alcohol and sweets. Triglyceride management involves a lifelong commitment to healthy lifestyle choices.

According to Dr. James Kenney, Ph.D., R.D., "If most people consumed a very low-fat diet with little animal protein, consisting mostly of natural foods, they would improve blood lipids, lose weight, and reduce the risk of heart disease."

If needed, drugs such as gemfibrozil (Lopid), fenofibrate (Tricor), and niacin, can also bring the triglyceride level down. For more information on drugs to reduce triglycerides, see Chapter 11. Check with your doctor about these drugs, of course.

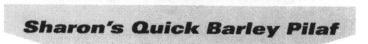

Sharon's Quick Barley Pilaf

A low-fat, high-fiber recipe

THIS RECIPE WAS inspired by a recipe from my friend Sharon Claessens, a healthy cook. Not only is it high in fiber—it contains 6 grams of dietary fiber per serving—but it is also high in soluble fiber, the type that lowers cholesterol.

¼ cup	pine nuts
1 tsp.	olive oil
4	scallions, thinly sliced
1	garlic clove, minced
2 cups	low-fat chicken broth
1 cup	quick-cooking barley
1	zucchini, diced
1	yellow squash, diced
1 tbs.	minced fresh parsley

Cook the pine nuts in olive oil over low heat until golden, 5 to 6 minutes, stirring occasionally. Watch the nuts, as they burn easily. Remove from the pan and set aside. Add the scallion and garlic, and cook, stirring, 1 minute. Add the chicken broth and bring to a boil. Stir in the barley. Return to a boil, reduce heat, cover, and simmer 5 minutes. Stir in the zucchini and yellow squash. Cover and simmer 7 minutes more. Stir in the parsley and pine nuts. Cover and remove from heat. Allow to set for at least 5 minutes. Serve.

❨ Yield: 4 servings ❩

Per serving: 174 calories, 28 g carbohydrates, 7 g protein, 4 g fat, 0 mg cholesterol, 6 g dietary fiber, 2 g soluble fiber, 62 mg sodium.

DIAGNOSIS: HIGH CHOLESTEROL

Blood Tests: Their Reliability and Understanding the Results

When people speak of *high cholesterol* or *low HDL* or *high triglycerides* or *high LDL,* what they mean is the blood levels of these various substances. Thus when, you schedule an annual checkup, you will be asked for a blood sample. The best time to take blood is early in the morning, after a twelve-hour fast, before eating breakfast.

Your level of triglycerides fluctuates up and down during the day. In the previous chapter, you learned that triglyceride levels are high immediately after a high-calorie, high-fat meal. So you wouldn't get an accurate reading of your triglycerides right after a meal. Triglyceride levels are also raised after drinking excessive amounts of alcohol, during sickness, and under stress.

This is why it is best to fast for a blood test. It is also best to have a second blood test to get an average of at least two tests.

How To Get a Good or Reliable Test

There are several types of tests that can be performed:

1. Blood test taken after a twelve-hour fast
2. Blood test taken and read without fasting
3. Home testing

In most physical checkups, a blood sample is taken from the arm and sent to a laboratory. Although nonfasting cholesterol tests used to be the norm, new guidelines issued by the National Cholesterol Education Program now recommend a fasting complete lipoprotein assessment to evaluate cholesterol levels. The results of the test, after a twelve-hour fast, include tryglycerides, total cholesterol, HDL cholesterol, LDL cholesterol, and a cholesterol/HDL ratio.

Ask for a copy of the blood test results from the doctor or the lab. The lab form will note what is optimal or in the normal range according to the individual testing lab report. Your cholesterol levels will be measured in milligrams per deciliter (mg/dL).

Lab Results:
Normal or Optimal Ranges

Triglycerides	lower than 150 mg/dL
Total Cholesterol	lower than 200 mg/dL
HDL Cholesterol	more than 40 mg/dL
LDL Cholesterol	100 mg/dL or lower
Cholesterol/HDL ratio	4.45 or lower

What Your Blood Test Results Mean

Most researchers and doctors agree that a total cholesterol level lower than 200 mg/dL is best. However, it has been found that for adults over 75 years of age, a total cholesterol level of 232 or above has a protective effect. Cholesterol metabolism is different as you age.

HDL levels above 60 mg/dL are considered especially beneficial and can offset another risk factor for coronary heart disease, according to the National Heart, Blood, and Lung Institute.

LDL numbers should be under 100 mg/dL, and triglycerides under 150 mg/dL.

If your test was done without fasting, then only the total cholesterol and the HDL values are usable. If your total cholesterol tested higher than 200 and your HDL lower than 40, then you should have the test redone and make sure you fast for 12 hours before the test.

If your results are high, you can start following the treatment guidelines of the National Cholesterol Education Program, as outlined in Chapter 6.

What Does the Chol/HDLC Ratio Mean?

When the total cholesterol value on the test results are divided by the HDL value, the result is the cholesterol/HDL ratio, sometimes written as CHOL/HDLC. The ratio should ideally be less than 4, and definitely between 3.6 and 6.4. In the past, this number was considered important, but new guidelines downplay the importance of this ratio, and most doctors do not check it when deciding on treatment.

At What Age Should You Have Your Cholesterol Tested?

As noted earlier, it's good to start having lipid tests at the age of twenty years. The National Heart, Lung, and Blood Institute recommends that everyone older than twenty have blood cholesterol levels checked at least once every five years, or more frequently, depending on their health or their doctor's wishes.

What the Numbers Mean

The **blood cholesterol numbers**, which apply to anyone over 20 years of age:

Blood Cholesterol Results:

DESIRABLE: Lower than 200 mg/dL
BORDERLINE-HIGH: 200–239 mg/dL
HIGH: 240 mg/dL and above

LDL Cholesterol Results:

OPTIMAL: Less than 100 mg/dL
ABOVE OPTIMAL: 100–129 mg/dL
BORDERLINE HIGH: 130–159 mg/dL
HIGH: 160–189 mg/dL
VERY HIGH: Above 190 mg/dL

HDL Cholesterol Results:

DESIRABLE: 60 mg/dL or higher
OPTIMAL: 40–59 mg/dL
RISK: Lower than 40 mg/dL

Triglyceride Results:

NORMAL: 150 mg/dL or lower
BORDERLINE-HIGH: 150–199 mg/dL
HIGH: 200–499 mg/dL
VERY HIGH: 500 mg/dL or higher

Source: National Cholesterol Education Program 2001

How About Homocysteine?

Another test that you may have done when you have blood drawn is the homocysteine (ho-mo-SIS-teen) level. There is evidence that the homocysteine level is linked to heart disease.

Homocysteine is a protein breakdown product that is found in the blood. When the blood of people with heart disease or blocked arteries was studied, it was found that the homocysteine level was high.

The homocysteine levels in healthy people are kept low by the presence of three B vitamins: folate, vitamin B_6, and vitamin B_{12}. If these vitamins are not available, the homocysteine level in the blood rises.

At this time it has not been proven that high homocysteine levels are a heart attack risk, but some doctors are recommending that their patients supplement their diets with these three B vitamins. Testing for homocysteine can be expensive, so doctors are not recommending it to everyone.

Researchers are not positive what the normal and high levels of homocysteine should be, but a homocysteine level over 16 micromoles per liter of blood is considered high, according to Dr. Paul Jacques, Acting Chief of Epidemiology at the Human Nutrition Research Center at Tufts.

Supplement Recommendations for the Three B Vitamins

Without heart disease:

➤ 400 mcg (micrograms) folate

➤ 3 mg B_6

➤ 6 mcg B_{12}

With heart disease:

➤ 400 mcg folate

➤ 4 mg B_6

➤ 8 mcg B_{12}

The following tables show some foods with these vitamins in them.

Folate (aim for 400 mcg per day)	
½ cup lentils	179
½ cup chickpeas	141
½ cup kidney beans	115

½ cup frozen spinach	102
1 cup General Mills Cheerios	100
1 cup Kellogg's Corn Flakes	100
1 cup Ronzoni spaghetti	100
6 oz. orange juice (from frozen concentrate)	82
½ cup frozen Brussels sprouts	79
½ cup frozen chopped broccoli	52
½ cup Minute Rice	40

B_6 mg

(aim for 3.0 mg a day, 4.0 mg a day if you have heart disease)

1 baked potato with skin	0.7
1 banana	0.7
1 cup Post Raisin Bran	0.7
3 oz. roasted light-meat chicken	0.5
3 oz. beef tenderloin	0.4
½ cup mashed sweet potato	0.4
½ Florida avocado	0.4
3 oz. lean roasted pork	0.4
3 oz. tuna (canned in water)	0.3
6 oz. canned vegetable juice cocktail	0.3
1 ear corn	0.2

B_{12} mcg

(aim for 6.0 mcg a day, 8.0 mcg daily if you have heart disease)
People with heart disease probably need a multivitamin supplement that contains enough B vitamins to meet the higher goal. B_{12} is found naturally only in foods of animal origin, although a number of breakfast cereals are fortified with it.

1⅓ cups General Mills Total	6.0
3 oz. tuna (canned in water)	2.5
3 oz. beef tenderloin	2.2
2 Atlantic sardines	2.0
3 frozen fish sticks	1.5
1 cup yogurt	1.0
1 cup skim milk	0.9

3 oz. broiled pork loin	0.9
1.6 oz. beef frankfurter	0.7
1 oz. Swiss cheese	0.5
3 oz. roasted light-meat chicken	0.3

And Now That You Have Your Test Results?

After you get your test results, your physician will go over them with you. If your LDL level is above 100 mg/dL, you will need a physical examination to check if there is a disease or condition that is elevating your cholesterol level. If there isn't, you and your physician will initiate a plan to get the level into the desirable range.

If your fasting test reveals that your total cholesterol is above 200, your risk for heart disease is increased. If you are in the "high" category, your risk is twice the risk of someone in the "desirable" category. You definitely need to do something if you are in the "high" category.

If you are in the "high" category and you have another risk factor for heart disease, it is even more important for you to take action now. For example, if your blood pressure is high and you have a high cholesterol level, you should look into starting to help yourself immediately.

Problems in Testing

Currently, when you are tested for possible heart problems, the total cholesterol, HDL, LDL, triglycerides, and homocysteine levels are usually checked. There are other substances in the blood that may give more reliable estimates of your heart disease risk, and in the future there may be standard tests for these substances as well. These include tests for cardiac enzymes, high-sensitivity C-reactive protein, and Lp(a).

One of the new tests measures the level of protein in cholesterol particles, or the **apolipoproteins.** Measuring LDL—the bad cholesterol— along with the apolipoprotein attached to the LDL, called apolipoprotein B (apo-B), was found to be more accurate in predicting a fatal heart attack than simply measuring the LDL alone. Apolipoprotein A1 (apo-A1) is attached to HDL and protects against heart attacks. This test seemed to be a better predictor of heart attacks when cholesterol levels were normal. You will most likely be hearing more about this test in the near future.

Home Tests

According to Dore Kottler, R.Ph., there are home cholesterol testing devices, but because of the high cost of the devices, sales have not been high. Also, she said most people would rather go to their doctor or lab and have blood taken than stick themselves.

There is a device which purportedly gives an accurate reading from a single drop of blood. The device is battery operated and costs $129.95. Six test strip refills are available for $21.95. There is a smart card replacement, which reads and stores your results and can even be used to send the results over the Internet to the doctor. More than one person can use the device as long as each person has the smart card. The device is available through a catalog at *www.intelihealth.com.* After getting to the site, go to "catalog," then "condition specific," then "heart and blood pressure," then "cholesterol monitor." The device can also be ordered by telephoning 1-800-988-1127.

Another home cholesterol meter called BioScanner 2000 can be ordered through Amazon.com or by checking *www.healthchecksystems.com.* It costs $149.95. It can also be ordered by telephoning 1-888-337-4684; for information call 718-339-6212. Try asking at your local pharmacy for more information.

CholesTrak is a twelve-minute cholesterol test kit approved by the Food and Drug Administration. A kit that includes the equipment for two tests costs $17.99. It is manufactured by AccuTech, LLC and should be available at neighborhood drug stores, including Albertsons, CVS, Eckerds, Longs, and Walgreen. You can learn more at *www.cholestrak.com*.

Greek Salad

A recipe high in folates, B_{12}, and B_6

2 tomatoes, quartered
1 cucumber, peeled and sliced
½ sweet red pepper, cored, seeded, and sliced
½ green pepper, cored, seeded, and sliced
5 scallions, thinly sliced (about ½ cup)
4 oz. crumbled feta cheese (or low-fat feta)
12–16 kalamata olives
½ head romaine lettuce, torn

Dressing:
3 tbs. red wine vinegar
2 cloves garlic, minced
½ tsp. dried oregano or 1 teaspoon fresh
⅛ tsp. black pepper
3 tbs. olive oil

1. In a large salad bowl, combine the tomatoes, cucumber, red and green pepper, scallions, feta cheese, and olives. Add the torn romaine.
2. Combine the dressing ingredients. Whisk together and pour over the salad ingredients. Toss and serve.

《 Yield: 4 servings 》

Per serving: 245 calories, 7 g protein, 13 g carbohydrates, 4 g dietary fiber, 1 g soluble fiber, 20 g fat, 11 g mono fat, 6 g sat fat, 25 mg cholesterol, 518 mg sodium. High in mono fat, vitamin A, thiamin, riboflavin, folate, B_6, B_{12}, calcium.

Are You at Risk?

If your total cholesterol and your LDL (Low Down Lousy) levels are high, you are at risk for heart disease. If you have high blood pressure, you are at risk for heart disease. If you smoke, you are at risk for heart disease. The more risks, the better your chances of having heart disease.

If you eat only white flour products and the only vegetable you eat are french fries, you are at risk. The more you expose yourself to these health hazards, the greater your chances of becoming ill.

If you want to live longer and healthier, you want your cholesterol level to be low. Right now if your blood cholesterol level is 200 or higher and your LDL is over 100, your doctor will take a second look. If your blood cholesterol level is 350 or more you *have* to do something. You are a heart attack waiting to happen. You are at the greatest risk if you have all three major heart disease risks factors, as listed on page 45.

New treatment guidelines for cholesterol were issued in May 2001 by the National Cholesterol Education Program, a division of the National Institutes of Health. The new guidelines focus on reducing LDL and recommend more intensive treatments.

The guidelines also emphasize better methods for identifying persons at high risk for heart disease. The emphasis in the new guidelines is preventing coronary heart disease in persons with multiple risk factors instead of waiting for a heart attack to occur.

So let's take a look at your own chances of developing heart disease:

The Three Major Heart Disease Risks

High cholesterol and high LDL

Smoking or daily exposure to smoke

High blood pressure (higher than 140/90 mmHg, or already on blood pressure medication)

Other risks are:

Genes: a family history of heart disease, especially occurring before age fifty-five in your father or before age sixty-five in your mother

Lack of physical activity

Being overweight

Poor diet: high fat, little fiber, minimal fruits and vegetables

Diabetes

Vascular disease: any disease of the blood vessels or the arteries and veins

Age: the older you are, the greater the risk

Low HDL levels: under 40 mg/dL

Look over the list above. How many risks do you have? Which risks are the ones you can do something about? The more risks you have, the more you will need to reduce some of those risks to avoid heart disease. Now let's see how you can estimate your overall risk for heart disease.

Estimate Your Ten-Year Risk for Developing Heart Disease

These risks and numbers were developed by the Heart, Lung, and Blood Institute using the risk factors included in an important long-term study of heart health called the Framingham study. The factors included are age, total cholesterol, HDL cholesterol, systolic blood pressure (top number), treatment for hypertension, and cigarette smoking. In addition, other major risks, such as family history, are factored in. It is designed for those adults over twenty years who do not have heart disease or diabetes.

To get your risk score, fill in the points, below. The numbers that you use to fill in your points come from the tables that follow. Find your numbers in the tables according to your age and sex, then fill in the blanks with your points.

For example, the first blank is for the age points. Don't put your chronological age in that blank. Put in the number next to your age that you find in the table on page 47.

Risk Score

	Points	
Age	_____	(from table p. 47)
Total cholesterol	_____	(from table p. 47–49)
High-density lipoprotein (HDL)	_____	(from table p. 49)
Systolic blood pressure	_____	(from table p. 50)
Cigarette smoking	_____	(from table p. 51)

Add all of the above numbers
for your total score   _____
            Percentage   _____

To find out what your risk for having a heart attack in the next ten years is, look at the last table and find your total score. You will find your percentage risk next to that number.

Age points

Find your age in the column on the left and look across to your points under "Male" or "Female." Fill in the number in the Risk Score line for age points.

Age	Male	Female
20–34	–9	–7
35–39	–4	–3
40–44	0	0
45–49	3	3
50–54	6	6
55–59	8	8
60–64	10	10
65–69	11	12
70–74	12	14
75–79	13	16

Total cholesterol points

If your total cholesterol is *less than 160 mg/dL* (from an average of at least two blood tests), then fill in a 0 on the risk score line for total cholesterol points.

If your total cholesterol is *from 160 to 199 mg/dL* (from an average of at least two blood tests), find your age in the left-hand column and then use the numbers under "Male" or "Female" to fill in the points on the risk score line for total cholesterol.

Age	Male	Female
20–39	4	4
40–49	3	3
50–59	2	2
60–69	1	1
70–79	0	1

Total cholesterol points

If your total cholesterol is *from 200 to 239 mg/dL* (from the average of at least two blood tests), find your age in the left-hand column and then use the number under "Male" or "Female" to fill in your points on the risk score line for total cholesterol.

Age	Male	Female
20–39	7	8
40–49	5	6
50–59	3	4
60–69	1	2
70–79	0	1

Total cholesterol points

If your total cholesterol is *from 240 to 279 mg/dL* (from the average of at least two blood tests), find your age in the left-hand hand column and then use the number under "Male" or "Female" to fill in your points on the risk score line for total cholesterol.

Age	Male	Female
20–39	9	11
40–49	6	8
50–59	4	5
60–69	2	3
70–79	1	2

Total cholesterol points

If your total cholesterol is *280 mg/dL or above* (from the average of at least two blood tests), find your age in the left-hand column and then use the number under "Male" or "Female" for your points on the risk score line for total cholesterol.

Age	Male	Female
20–39	11	13
40–49	8	10
50–59	5	7
60–69	3	4
70–79	1	2

HDL score

Your HDL should be from the average of at least two blood tests. Find your HDL score in the column on the left, then use the number under "Male" or "Female" to fill in your point score in the risk score line for HDL.

HDL	Male	Female
60+	−1	−1
50–59	0	0
40–49	1	1
Lower than 40	2	2

Blood pressure score

If you *are not on blood pressure medication,* look down the left-hand column for your systolic blood pressure number (top number of your blood pressure), then use the points that are under "Male" or "Female" to fill in your point score in the risk score line for blood pressure.

BP	Male	Female
Lower than 120	0	0
120–129	0	1
130–139	1	2
140–159	1	3
160+	2	4

Blood pressure score

If you *are taking medication for blood pressure,* look down the left-hand column for your systolic blood pressure number (top number of your blood pressure), then use the points under "Male" or "Female" to fill in your point score in the risk score line for blood pressure.

BP	Male	Female
Lower than 120	0	0
120–129	1	3
130–139	2	4
140–159	2	5
160+	3	6

Smoking status

If you have not smoked one cigarette in the past month, give
yourself a score of 0. If you had one or more cigarettes in the
past month then use this table. Check your age in the left-
hand column, then look across for your score under "Male"
or "Female." Write that number on the risk score line for
smoking.

Age	Male	Female
20–39	8	9
40–49	5	7
50–59	3	4
60–69	1	2
70–79	1	1

Ten-Year Risk

Use the table below to find your ten-year risk for developing
heart disease with the number you got as a total score. Adding
the numbers you got for age, cholesterol, HDL, blood pressure,
and smoking, find your total score in the column on the left
then look across under the "Male" or "Female" column to find
your percentage risk for developing heart disease in the next
ten years.

Total Score	Risk for Males	Risk for Females
Less than 0	Less than 1%	Less than 1%
0	1%	Less than 1%
1–4	1%	Less than 1%
5–6	2%	Less than 1%
7	3%	Less than 1%
8	4%	Less than 1%
9	5%	1%
10	6%	1%
11	8%	1%
12	10%	1%
13	12%	2%

Total Score	Risk for Males	Risk for Females
14	16%	2%
15	20%	3%
16	25%	4%
17	30%	5%
18	30%	6%
19	30%	8%
20	30%	11%
21	30%	14%
22	30%	17%
23	30%	22%
24	30%	27%
25 or more	30%	30%

Recommendations for the Highest Risk

1. If your risk is 20 percent or more and you have diabetes, already have coronary heart disease, or have two or more risk factors, your immediate goal is to lower your LDL to less than 100 mg/dL. Out of 100 people in this category, 20 will develop coronary heart disease or have a heart attack in the next 10 years.
2. If you already have two or more risk factors, you need to make lifestyle changes to reduce your LDL levels. The first steps should be to exercise and limit your fat intake.
3. If you have no risk factors or one risk factor but your LDL level is above 160, try lifestyle changes first. If you have an LDL level of over 190, seek advice from your doctor, who may advise medication.

The following chapters discuss lowering your risks in more detail, particularly with lifestyle changes.

Savory Chicken and Vegetable Stew

A high-fiber, low-cholesterol, and low-saturated fat recipe

2 tbs.	olive oil
1	onion, chopped
1 lb.	chicken breast, boned, skinned, and cut into chunks
5 cups	low-fat, low-sodium chicken broth
1 cup	long-grain brown rice
2	carrots, peeled and cut into chunks
1 can (15 oz.)	low-sodium pinto beans, if not low-sodium, (rinse and drain)
1 tsp.	cumin seeds
1 tsp.	dried oregano or 2 tsp. fresh
10 oz. package	fresh spinach, rinsed and coarsely chopped

1. In a large pot, heat the oil, then add the onion and chicken. Stir and cook until the onions are softened.

2. Add the broth, rice, carrots, beans, cumin, and oregano and bring to a boil. Lower the heat, cover, and cook for 40 minutes or until the rice is tender.

3. Add the spinach, re-cover, and cook for 2 minutes. Stir to combine, and serve.

❪ **Yield: 6 servings** ❫

Per serving: 348 calories, 30 g protein, 39 g carbohydrates, 7.5 g fat, 1.4 g sat fat, 7 g dietary fiber, 1 g soluble fiber, 45 mg cholesterol, 238 mg sodium.

PART 2:

High Cholesterol and You

How to Lower Cholesterol
or Keep it Low

One of the best precautions you can take to prevent heart disease or atherosclerosis is to keep your cholesterol below 200 mg/dL and to keep your LDL (Low Down Lousy) cholesterol below 100 mg/dL. These are current recommendations based on research studies.

Red Flags

Take a serious look at your lifestyle *if your cholesterol and LDL are high and:*

you have diabetes. You should be treated as if you already had a heart attack.

you have many risk factors but no previous heart attack, stroke, or coronary heart disease.

you have less than 40 mg/dL of HDL, the "healthy" cholesterol.

To treat elevated blood cholesterol, specifically the LDL (Low Down Lousy) cholesterol, the newest guidelines of the National Cholesterol Education Program emphasizes intensified use of:

nutrition
physical activity
weight control

These newest guidelines advise a *Therapeutic Lifestyle Changes* (TLC) treatment plan that includes a cholesterol-lowering diet (the TLC diet). According to the National Cholesterol Education Program, one-third of U.S. adults (about 65 million people) should have dietary therapy. These guidelines were developed by a panel of twenty-seven members and consultants and reviewed by more than forty medical and health organizations. The guidelines are also known as the Adult Treatment Panel III.

The TLC Diet Guidelines

To lower LDL and cholesterol, the diet should include:

- ➤ less than 7 percent of calories from saturated fat
- ➤ less than 200 mg of dietary cholesterol
- ➤ up to 35 percent of daily calories from total fat
  - polyunsaturated fat can provide 10 percent of daily calories
  - monounsaturated fats can provide up to 20 percent of total calories
- ➤ the use of foods rich in soluble fiber to boost the diet's LDL-lowering power (10 to 25 g per day)

The guidelines also address drug therapy. According to the National Cholesterol Education Program, if all persons with cholesterol levels high enough to warrant drug therapy were identified and treated, the number of adults taking cholesterol-lowering drugs would go up to 36 million. Drugs do have side effects, so keep that in mind before quickly choosing drug therapy.

Try Nutrition First

Changing your diet has the most influence on LDL, so *eliminate some fat, especially trans fat and saturated fat, from your diet.* More about modifying your diet is explained in Chapters 8 and 9.

Does omitting all animal products and cholesterol from the diet make it a low-fat diet?

No, because there is fat in vegetable oils and hidden fat in baked goods. You don't want to eliminate all oils because you do need some. You can eat up to 35 percent oil/fat, according to the new guidelines. Just try to make them unsaturated and without trans fat.

Potato chips may have no cholesterol or animal fat, but they are usually high in fat. Peanut butter has no cholesterol and no animal fat, but it is high in fat. It can be eaten in moderation because it is high in the monounsaturated "good" fat.

Margarine can have no cholesterol but can be high in fat and also trans fat. Read the labels. If a food has 3 grams of fat per serving, or less, it is low in fat.

Try Exercise Next

Ideally your cholesterol and your LDL cholesterol will start going down when you start reducing the fat in your diet. Just remember that the cholesterol numbers may be an indicator of heart disease risk, but they don't tell you what the underlying cause is. Think of the speedometer in your car. If it goes up to 100, it's an indication that your car is going too fast—but it's not the cause. The cause of your high cholesterol may be *too little exercise*. The benefits of excercise are discussed further in Chapter 7.

Try Weight Loss

After trying exercise or more exercise, the next step you can take is to *lose some weight*. For many people, avoiding sugar, white flour (and anything made with it), and fried foods (especially deep-fried foods such as french fries or potato chips), is a way to omit unnecessary calories and lose a few pounds.

Cut Back on Saturated Fat

If lowering your fat or cholesterol intake doesn't help you lose weight or improve your cholesterol scores, then *cut back on saturated fat.*

Reducing your cholesterol intake lowers your risk of heart disease, but it has less impact on blood cholesterol levels than cutting back on saturated fat. Saturated fat and trans fat boost your blood cholesterol level more than anything else in your diet.

Add Soluble Fiber

Adding soluble fiber (Chapter 9 lists sources of soluble fiber) and more fruits and vegetables is the next step to a healthier diet and the way to lower your cholesterol and become healthier. Here is an instance in which eating more will lower your blood cholesterol level, particularly the LDL level. According to Dr. James Kenney, Ph.D., "For every one or two grams of soluble fiber you consume daily, you will lower your LDL by 1 percent."

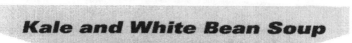

Kale and White Bean Soup

A cholesterol-lowering recipe

THIS HEARTY SOUP is a high-soluble fiber recipe that will help you lower your cholesterol. For faster preparation, use 2 cans (15 oz.) of no-salt white beans.

¾ cup	dried white or Michigan beans (2 cups cooked)
3½ cups	water
1 tbs.	olive oil
1	medium onion, peeled and chopped
2 cloves	garlic, peeled and minced
1 stalk	celery, finely chopped
1	carrot, peeled and finely chopped
1	bay leaf
4 cups	water
8 ounces	kale, washed and coarsely chopped, leaves only
1 tablespoon	fresh dill
	Freshly ground black pepper (garnish)

1. Soak the beans in a covered pot, in enough boiling water to cover, for one hour. Drain the beans and add to a 3-quart pot with 3½ cups water. Bring to a boil, lower the heat, cover, and continue cooking at a slow boil until the beans are tender, about 1 hour.
2. Heat the oil in a 4-quart pot. Saute the onion, garlic, celery, and carrot on low until softened, 10 to 15 minutes. Add the bay leaf and 4 cups of water and bring to a boil. Lower the heat, cover, and cook for 20 minutes. Add the drained, cooked beans, chopped kale, and dill. Cover and continue to cook for 10 minutes. Remove the bay leaf. Serve garnished with black pepper.

{ Yield: 6 servings }

Per serving: 131 calories, 7 g protein, 21 g carbohydrate, 3 g fat, 2 g mono fat, 0 mg cholesterol, 5 g dietary fiber, 1.6 g soluble fiber, 28 mg sodium.

Try Different Changes

Try different lifestyle changes to see what works best for you. Losing extra weight, quitting smoking, and becoming more physically active may help boost your HDL (Heart's De-Lite or "good") cholesterol level. Another result of this healthy living is lower blood pressure. It's a win/win situation.

Can I Include Any Saturated Fat or Cholesterol in My Diet?

There is still some controversy over how low the amount of saturated fat and cholesterol in your diet has to go to affect your blood cholesterol and your risk of heart disease.

For example, researchers have studied the Masai tribes in Africa who eat only red meat and drink blood and several quarts of whole milk a day. And they don't have heart disease. However, they do *exercise* and they are *thin*.

The editor of the Egg Nutriton Center newsletters *Nutrition Close-Up* and *Nutrition Realities*, Donald J. McNamara, Ph.D., feels that lowering the amount of cholesterol in the diet from 300 mg to 200 mg puts the "wrong emphasis in the wrong direction." *If the saturated fat content of your diet is already low,* then lowering your dietary cholesterol intake will not benefit you much, according to the center's newsletter. Even though a spokesperson for the Egg Nutrition Center might be considered biased, I agree with Dr. McNamara.

Eggs: How Bad Are They?

Eggs have gotten a bad rap, according to Egg Nutrition Center spokesperson Dr. McNamara. "The evidence against eating eggs is weak. After 30 years of being maligned for its supposed role in raising blood cholesterol levels, eggs are making a comeback, thanks to mounting scientific evidence refuting this myth."

In 2000, the American Heart Association increased their egg recommendation from three to four egg yolks to seven egg yolks per week. Your diet should be low in saturated fat and no more than 30 percent calories from fat for this to be recommended.

It appears that eggs can be safely consumed, in moderation of course. If the American Heart Association quietly upped the recommended intake of yolks, they must feel that eating eggs in moderation is okay. Make an omelette with an egg and some egg substitute if you like. Nobody really needs a three-egg omelette! A three-egg plain omelette without ham or cheese added would contain about 263 calories, 18 grams of fat, and 531 mg of cholesterol

Eggs do have their benefits. We used to eat eggs because they were easy to digest. We fed eggs to children as a great source of protein. Eggs are low in fat and high in choline, and they contain the highest-quality and least-expensive protein in the supermarket as well as a wide spectrum of vitamins and minerals. Eggs also contain phytochemicals (see Chapter 8) lutein and zeaxanthin, two carotenoids that are deposited in the retina and protect against macular degeneration.

Can I Reduce
Cholesterol by Myself?

I asked Dr. Norman Sarachek, a heart specialist, how much time he allowed patients to try to lower their cholesterol levels on their own before he prescribed a drug. He answered, "One day." In his experience, not one patient of his has been able to change his or her lifestyle no matter how much time he allowed them. "Drugs work better and faster," he said.

However, if you want to avoid drugs and their side effects, see what you can do first before taking medication. There are doctors who *do* have patients who successfully lower their LDL (Low Down Lousy) cholesterol without medication. You may want to try to see what you can do. It can happen. There are several effective medications for lowering cholesterol, and these are an option in conjunction with lifestyle changes. Medications are discussed in Chapter 11.

How Best to Lower Your LDL Cholesterol

According to the *Communicating Food For Health* newsletter (copyright *www.foodandhealth.com*), the following are good ways to reduce LDL. If you can adhere to these ten recommendations for three to four weeks, your LDL should go down 20 to 50 percent. Can you do it?

- **Eat foods high in fiber, especially soluble fiber,** which is found in beans, fruits, root vegetables, oats, barley, corn, rice bran, apples, strawberries, and flax. Your goal is 10 to 25 grams of soluble fiber every day.
- **Eat small meals.** About 6 to 8 per day is better than 1 to 2 large meals.
- **Eat nonfat dairy products.** They are best since they are lower in saturated fat.
- **Get 30 minutes of moderate exercise almost every day, which will raise your HDL.** Or walk at least 2 to 3 miles per day 5 to 6 days a week.
- **Limit the saturated fat you eat** by basing your meals on beans, vegetables, fruit, and whole grains with a

minimum of animal protein foods. This would be about 10 to 11 grams of saturated fat daily, which includes using nonfat dairy, fish, and egg whites. Replace butter with vegetable spreads, such as hummus, or with olive oil.

- **Avoid foods with trans fat.** This is the fat noted on labels as *partially hydrogenated vegetable oil.* It is often found in fried foods and processed foods such as crackers, baked goods, and desserts.
- **Limit your daily cholesterol intake** to 200 mg.
- **Lose weight** if you are overweight. This will raise your HDL cholesterol and lower your total cholesterol.
- **Include soy protein** in your diet. Including 25 grams of soy protein per day helps lower cholesterol when it is part of a heart-healthy diet.
- **Limit your intake of sugar.** This should lower triglycerides, increase weight loss, and help lower your LDL.
- **Consider using sterol- and stanol-rich margarines** (see next section). Plant sterols are also found in beans, nuts, and seeds.

Functional Foods: Sterol- and Stanol-Rich Margarine

Scientists have come up with a product that you *add* to your diet to help lower your cholesterol. Especially for those who like to use a lot of margarine or butter on bread or vegetables, this functional food may be the answer.

A functional food is one that has been formulated in a food laboratory to help prevent some illness or disease. For example, there are bottled waters that have added vitamins. Some manufacturers think plain water should be enhanced with vitamins to give it more reason to be consumed (and also so they can charge more for it). You might find eggs enhanced with omega-3 fatty acids, or orange juice with calcium added to help prevent osteoporosis. Look around and you will see more and more of these functional foods.

Can You Give Up Margarine or Butter?

If you like butter or margarine and eat a lot—let's say 2 tablespoons of butter or margarine a day—and you don't want to give it up, you might want to consider Benecol, made from stanols, or Take Control, made from sterols. These margarines contain a fatlike substance that actually lowers your cholesterol by blocking the absorption of cholesterol in the intestine. The Benecol label suggests you eat 2 to 3 tablespoons a day to reduce your LDL up to 14 percent and your total cholesterol up to 10 percent. If your total cholesterol is 230, and you used this margarine regularly, your cholesterol could drop to 207 in two weeks. If you stopped eating the margarine, your cholesterol would go back up.

Here are some points to consider:

- Take Control and Benecol come in regular and light.
- The first ingredient in both margarines is canola oil.
- Calories are about 45 calories per tablespoon for the Benecol light.
- Recipes for Benecol (on their web site) say it can be used for baking, cooking, and frying.
- Take Control advertises that 2 tablespoons a day will lower your LDL by 17 percent.
- The effect of these margarines depends on how high your cholesterol is to begin with. They work best when the diet is low in saturated fat and cholesterol.
- They are more than double the price of most margarines.

You can find out more about Take Control at *www.takecontrol.com* or by calling 800-735-3554; or about Benecol at *www.benecol.com* or by calling 888-benecol.

Margarine Or Butter?

What should you use? Some margarines advertise no trans fat, but they add saturated fat, which is just as bad as the partially hydrogenated fat they replace. Tub margarines are better in that the first ingredient can be water or an oil—for example, a healthier canola oil.

Again, as with any food, read the ingredient labels. Choose a margarine with as little saturated fat and trans fat as possible. If you substitute margarine for butter, choose a soft margarine that is trans-fat free. In a study done at the U.S. Department of Agriculture's Human Nutrition Research Center in Beltsville, Maryland, where forty-six men and women ate butter, tub margarine, and trans-fat free tub margarine, the margarines improved blood cholesterol levels. And the trans-free soft margarine was better than the regular soft margarine, although only by a small amount.

What Is Best for You?

Medications, diet, functional foods, and exercise all help to lower cholesterol. Which is best for you?

Well, some things are always going to be good, no matter how things change. You might get confused about whether you are doing the right things or eating the right foods when you read the newspaper or listen to television.

These things are good for you:

- Exercise
- Maintaining a healthy weight
- Not smoking

- Drinking water
- Eating. Eating is good, it's just that *what* and *how much* can change when you're trying to reduce your cholesterol. But there are some things that remain good for you:

> **Fruits and vegetables: fresh, steamed, baked, boiled, roasted**
> **Oatmeal**
> **Brown rice**
> **A cup of freshly brewed hot coffee**
> **A glass of red wine with a meal**
> **Hot or iced tea**
> **A piece of dark chocolate occasionally**

When you add a new healthy practice, talk to your health care professional about when to take a follow-up blood test to see how you are doing.

EXERCISE AND
STRESS REDUCTION

If you get a diagnosis of a high total cholesterol or LDL (Low Down Lousy) level, or a low HDL (Heart's De-Lite) level, you may wonder what the best corrective path is for you. What should you do? What will you actually do? Cardiologist Dr. Norman Sarachek never had a patient who could change his or her lifestyle. Is that you?

If you smoke, can you stop smoking? Cutting out that habit will raise your good, or HDL, cholesterol. Don't frequent places where smokers gather either. Your HDL also responds to exercise and weight loss, And if your LDL is too high, well, that responds best to a change of diet.

Exercise

Exercise is a proven way to lower your cholesterol, raise your HDL, lower your LDL, and improve your health in general. Exercise will help you lose weight and tone your muscles. More calories are expended, and you will look and feel better.

The benefits of exercise are constantly confirmed. About thirty minutes a day produces a healthier you. Those who exercise have lower rates of heart disease, quicker recovery rates if they do have a heart attack, optimal blood pressure, higher HDL cholesterol, less instances of diabetes, more lean muscle mass, less instances of osteoporosis, less pain from arthritis, less stress, and less depression. They live longer and feel better. So why are we becoming a nation of couch potatoes?

To lower heart disease risk, a recent study revealed, you don't have to exercise vigorously. For middle-aged women, walking about one hour a week with a pace of 3 miles per hour resulted in a 50 percent reduction in heart disease risk.

When women chose walking—which seems to be the most common exercise choice among women—the duration of the walk had a greater effect on lowering heart disease risk compared with the intensity. You don't have to power walk, but walking for a half hour to an hour at a time rather than just ten minutes now and then is what you want to achieve.

There are four major risk factors for heart disease—smoking, excess body weight, high blood pressure, and high blood cholesterol. The researchers noted that exercise was especially important in lowering the risk for smokers and those with normal blood pressure. So get out and move.

Why Don't You Exercise?

Are These Your Excuses?

- I will only walk with my dog, and my husband walked the dog earlier
- I don't like to walk in the dark, and nighttime is the only free time I have.
- I don't like to walk.
- I don't like to walk alone.
- I don't want to join a fitness center.
- I have an exercise bicycle, and I don't use it.
- I don't have time.

The excuses go on and on. Remember: It is your *life* that is involved here!

Pick a Type of Exercise
That You Like and Will Do

Check what is available in your town. Aerobics classes can be fun and free at the local Y, high school, or church. Swimming may appeal to you. Swimming and aerobics are a great combination. A popular exercise class is the Balanced Fitness class, which involves the use of a "stability ball," which is an oversized, superstrength beach ball that you work with as you do a series of movements.

According to cardiologist Dr. Stephen Shore, "A well-balanced program includes three kinds of exercise":

1. Cardiovascular exercise for your heart, such as walking or swimming
2. Resistance training or weight training for strength
3. Stretching for balance and flexibility

You've heard that you should park as far away from the building as is feasible to get in those extra steps and burn those calories. Walk up the stairs. Wash the floor on your hands and knees to get in the stretching exercises. Lift food cans, equivalent to one-pound weights, and walk around the house a bit more. In an article in *Cooking Light* magazine, JoAnna Lund, a cookbook author, said she found if she walks "downstairs through the hallway, the library, pass through my study, into my family room, over to the cookstove, and back up to the hall 14 times, that's a mile." And she does that a few times a day. Put on a pedometer and see how many miles you can walk in a day.

Need more ideas? Weight training, yoga, or step aerobics? How about cardio-kickboxing? Running? Hiking? Cycling? Pilates, jazzercise, Taebo, spinning? Golf, tennis, bowling? Skiing? Ice skating? Roller Skating? In-line skating? Boxing? Dancing? Swing or Country Western lessons? Square dancing?

According to the U.S. Department of Health and Human Services, you should start out slowly but work up to 30 minutes a day, which can be 10 minutes at a time, done three times. But keep working at it. Holly McCord in her book *The Peanut Butter Diet* lists "vitamin X" (for exercise) as necessary for health. She recommends forty-five minutes every day.

Exercise will:

- make you feel more energetic
- help you lose weight and control your appetite
- help you sleep better
- lower your chance for diabetes
- lower your chance for a stroke
- lower your blood pressure
- improve your blood cholesterol levels

I find that setting aside time first thing in the morning works best for me. That is a good beginning to the day. I walk outside in the early morning. I like being outside in any weather, and I started by walking for five minutes out, and then back.

Little by little I walked a bit farther, giving myself a goal, such as a drugstore, shopping center, or a bank that was about a half mile away. If it was raining, I watched an exercise show in the early morning and exercised along with the host. I didn't have the stamina in the beginning to do the complete half hour, but eventually I did and even had the stamina to work through the advertisements. I was amazed at myself. Then I took my walking/running shoes to work and walked at lunch, walking at least a mile. I used break time and invited other colleagues to come along. Walking and talking business meetings makes the work fun.

Other ideas to get you going and adding activity to your daily routine are as follows:

- Ride your stationary bike while watching TV or reading the paper

- ▶ Work out along with an exercise video
- ▶ Keep your hand weights near the telephone and use them during your telephone conversations
- ▶ Jump rope
- ▶ Garden
- ▶ Rake leaves

My eighty-six-year-old neighbor rakes leaves every day—during the season, of course. She finds other outdoor activity to do at other times: planting, hoeing around the plants, weeding, cutting flowers, and just walking around and admiring the garden.

Marty's Story

Imagine that you have always exercised; then you have your cholesterol tested, and it is 250. You're shocked. You say, "But I exercise!" That is what happened to Marty. During his twenties he weighed about 128 pounds at 5'8" and ran at least 65 miles a week during marathon training.

As the years went by, he continued to run, but his weight slowly rose. By the time he was 50, he weighed 152. Marty is still running 6 days a week, a total of about 35 miles. He takes a break on Mondays by walking for about 40 minutes, then on Tuesday, Wednesday, Thursday, and Friday, he runs for 30 to 40 minutes. Saturday he does a shorter run, and Sunday he runs for longer, about 1½ to 2 hours.

When he discovered that his cholesterol was 250 and he had gained 24 pounds over the years, he decided it was time to review his habits. He continued to exercise as he had, but he cut down his food intake. By cutting portions—especially bread, pasta, and potatoes—and increasing fruit and vegetable consumption, he lost 12 pounds. Now at 140 pounds at age 52, he feels better and was delighted to find that his cholesterol had dropped to 197. His HDL is an excellent 64, his LDL is 118, and his triglycerides are a very low 70.

By losing some of the weight that he had added over the years, Marty was able to lower his total cholesterol and lower his heart disease risk with the high HDL. He has his cholesterol checked once a year to keep it under control.

Stress Reduction

To reduce your chances of a heart attack, you should lessen the stress in your life. Release the tension in ways that will benefit you, especially if you eat or smoke to relieve stress.

In a study performed several years ago, it was found that the men with the highest cholesterol levels were those who repressed their anxiety. If you can vent your anger in a way that doesn't involve violence or shouting, such as through physical activity, that should help your health.

Some good ways to help fight anxiety—other than exercise—are massage therapy, biofeedback, and aromatherapy. There are all kinds of massage; like hot stone, you could get a flotation wrap, mud wrap, or oil wrap, shiatsu, reiki, and reflexology. Or how about a foot soak? Herbal bath? Jacuzzi or whirlpool? Hydrotherapy? Mineral bath, a bath surrounded by scented candles? T'ai chi, Qigong, rolfing? Steam room, sauna? Hair styling? Manicure? Facials? Pedicure? Relaxation techniques? Partnered relaxation? Mind and body classes? Mall walking and shopping? Playing with a pet? Deep breathing? Play a relaxation tape. Take a nap. Take a lunch break. Have a cup of herbal tea. Play music. Learn to play a musical instrument. Read a book. Buy a magazine. Take your phone outside to speak in the garden. Take your laptop outside and work on the patio. See a movie. Meditate. Pray. Anything that allows you to sit with your mind wandering and unfocused is helpful.

Scott James' Story

Scott James was working in a standing, walking, and lifting job at a scrap metal yard. At close to 5 feet 11 inches tall, and

49 years of age, he weighed more than he had ever weighed, which he realized by the waist size on his pants.

His wife was into health and diet, exercise, watching her weight, and cooking foods for herself that were low in fat. She was going to a nutrition consultant who helped her with recipes and menus. Dinners were usually fish, skinless chicken breasts, and salads. But Scott wanted meat and potatoes, so she made two meals every night for dinner: one low-fat meal for her and one high-fat and high-cholesterol meal for him.

Just before the December holidays that year, he developed a bad back, and on a particularly painful day, his wife suggested that he see a doctor. "Maybe he can give you a shot or pill that will help," she said. So when Scott went to the family doctor, who had not seen him for several years, the doctor was shocked at Scott's weight and suggested he have a complete blood work-up. His cholesterol level was of particular importance to the doctor, who knew that Scott's father had recently had bypass surgery.

Scott turned out to have a cholesterol level of 329 mg/dL and a weight of 202 pounds, more than had thought possible on both counts. Scott's weight in his late teens was a comfortable 165 pounds.

So Scott went home and conferred with his wife and said she shouldn't make two meals anymore; he would eat whatever she ate. She had been losing weight continuously.

He started exercising. Almost every day he walked on the treadmill for 10 miles at a comfortable rate of 4.2 miles an hour. He went to a personal trainer and worked with the trainer on strength training and stretching, using the Nautilus® and free weights about one hour a week, or even two hours a week if he had the time.

He didn't go back to the doctor, but he gave blood occasionally, and when he did, his blood cholesterol was checked, so he knew the numbers were going down.

He is eating more healthily now, taking a vitamin C supplement, a daily multivitamin supplement, and a pill containing cholestin, which he purchases at the health food store on the advice of the proprietor . Although, I don't think it is generally a good idea to get your health information from someone who sells a product, this pill, made from red yeast rice, purports to "support a healthy cholesterol." According to the Food and Drug Administration, it is derived from the same substance as the drug lovastatin. Note: taking this would have the same side effects as the statins, so blood tests monitoring liver enzymes should be checked regularly by a physician. I did suggest this to Scott.

Scott James is now 51 years old and has lost 42 pounds. His total cholesterol is 179 mg/dL.

This complete lifestyle change did help Scott. He feels much better, is back to his fighting weight, and looks much trimmer, and healthier. And his back is fine, too.

DIET AND WEIGHT LOSS

Lose Weight and Lower Your Cholesterol

Exercise and stress reduction to raise your HDL (Heart's De-Lite) cholesterol level is a beginning. To have the most impact on the LDL (Low Down Lousy) cholesterol, you need to either lose weight or change the types and portions of foods you eat. You might try eating smaller but healthy meals more frequently during the day. Look toward improving your eating habits. Try substituting good fats (monounsaturated and omega-3) for bad fats (saturated). Eat more fruits and vegetables. You can try different approaches to see what works best for you.

Losing weight—even 10 percent of your weight—will help lower your total cholesterol and in particular your LDL levels. If you are at your best weight, then you have to change the types of foods you are eating.

You probably know what your best or healthiest weight should be. If not, you can use the body mass index (BMI) to assess your healthiest weight. BMI is a relationship between height and weight. Overweight adults (18 years or older) with a BMI of higher than 25 are at risk for heart disease. Following is a BMI chart you can use to determine your own BMI:

Height (Feet and Inches)

Weight (Pounds)	5'0"	5'1"	5'2"	5'3"	5'4"	5'5"	5'6"	5'7"	5'8"	5'9"	5'10"	5'11"	6'0"	6'1"	6'2"	6'3"	6'4"
100	20	19	18	18	17	17	16	16	15	15	14	14	14	13	13	12	12
105	21	20	19	19	18	17	17	16	16	16	15	15	14	14	13	13	13
110	21	21	20	19	19	18	18	17	17	16	16	15	15	15	14	14	13
115	22	22	21	20	20	19	19	18	17	17	17	16	16	15	15	14	14
120	23	23	22	21	21	20	19	19	18	18	17	17	16	16	15	15	15
125	24	24	23	22	21	21	20	20	19	18	18	17	17	16	16	16	15
130	25	25	24	23	22	22	21	20	20	20	19	19	18	18	17	17	16
135	26	26	25	24	23	22	22	21	21	20	19	19	18	18	17	17	16
140	27	26	26	25	24	23	23	22	21	21	20	20	19	18	18	17	17
145	28	27	27	26	25	24	23	23	22	21	21	20	20	19	19	18	18
150	29	28	27	27	26	25	24	23	23	22	22	21	20	20	19	19	18
155	30	29	28	27	27	26	25	24	24	23	22	22	21	20	20	19	19
160	31	30	29	28	27	27	26	25	24	24	23	22	22	21	21	20	19
165	32	31	30	29	28	27	27	26	25	24	24	23	22	22	21	21	20
170	33	32	31	30	29	28	27	27	26	25	24	24	23	22	22	21	21
175	34	33	32	31	30	29	28	27	27	26	25	24	24	23	22	22	21
180	35	34	33	32	31	30	29	28	27	27	26	25	24	24	23	22	22
185	36	35	34	33	32	31	30	29	28	27	27	26	25	24	24	23	23
190	37	36	35	34	33	32	31	30	29	28	27	26	26	25	24	24	23
195	38	37	36	35	33	32	31	31	30	29	28	27	26	26	25	24	24
200	39	38	37	35	34	33	32	31	30	30	29	28	27	26	26	25	24
205	40	39	37	36	35	34	33	32	31	30	29	29	28	27	26	26	25
210	41	40	38	37	36	35	34	33	32	31	30	29	28	28	27	26	26
215	42	41	39	38	37	36	35	34	33	32	31	30	29	28	28	27	26
220	43	42	40	39	38	37	36	34	33	32	32	31	30	29	28	27	27
225	44	43	41	40	39	37	38	35	34	33	32	31	31	30	29	28	27
230	45	43	42	41	39	38	37	36	35	34	33	32	31	30	30	29	28
235	46	44	43	42	40	39	38	37	36	35	34	33	32	31	30	29	29
240	47	45	44	43	41	40	39	38	36	35	34	33	33	32	31	30	29
245	48	46	45	44	42	41	40	38	37	36	35	34	33	32	31	31	30
250	49	47	46	44	43	42	40	39	38	37	36	35	34	33	32	31	30

☐ Underweight   ☐ Weight Appropriate   ☐ Overweight   ☐ Obese

Source: The National Institutes of Health, NHLBI Clinical Guidelines on Overweight and Obesity, June 1998.

The frequency of meals can also make a difference. According to a recent study, if you eat one or two large meals a day, your cholesterol levels will be higher than those of people who spread their meals out over the day. Eating the same amount of food divided into six meals lowered not only total cholesterol levels but also LDL levels.

The American Dietetic Association recommends trying to lower your cholesterol through diet: "Your diet is an important factor in controlling cholesterol. A healthful low-fat eating plan, combined with regular physical activity, is key to heart health." In fact, as noted earlier, the new National Cholesterol Education Program guidelines say that one in three Americans need to make dietary changes to lower their risk for heart disease.

So what changes can you make to your diet to make it healthier? Let's talk about what you should eat.

Start With Soluble Fiber

Change No. 1. Choose foods high in soluble fiber, such as oatmeal, beans and peas, barley, and fruits and vegetables such as apples, oranges, and carrots.

The soluble fiber in foods (see table in Chapter 9) forms a gel similar to what you find surrounding the beans in a can of kidney beans. Once it gets into the intestine, that gel-like substance traps the cholesterol and keeps it from getting into your body. The soluble fiber isn't absorbed but passes out in the stool and takes the cholesterol with it. Studies have shown that those who get the most soluble fiber in their diet have the least risk for heart disease.

To lower your LDL, your food choices are key. Studies have shown that high—soluble fiber oatmeal helps to lower LDL cholesterol without lowering HDL.

Oatmeal

Having oatmeal for breakfast is a good way to start. Some folks happily tell me that they have started with the little presweetened and flavored packages of oatmeal that are added to water. This is a good way to *begin*. Read the labels and compare the amounts of dietary fiber and soluble fiber in various types of breakfast oatmeals. You will find that the less processed oats have more soluble fiber and fewer calories.

Mothers who give those dry round oat cereals to their children as snacks are starting them out in a good way. For every cup of Cheerios, you are getting 3 grams of dietary fiber and 1 gram of soluble fiber. Read and compare oats and oatmeal Nutrition Facts labels.

Apples

"An apple a day keeps the doctor away." It looks as if there is a lot of truth to that adage. Putting out a bowl of apples for the family may help them to eat apples. Try quartering an apple, spreading the quarters with peanut butter, and adding them to a lunch box. Cut an apple into a fruit salad. Make a microwave applesauce. Prepare a baked apple. Make the following recipe for Cranberry Apple Dumplings. It's a little high in fat but easy, and everyone will *eat* that apple. I want to stress that this recipe is not for everyday, but a special dessert. Most important, all the fat is in the pie dough, so you can omit that and make a plain baked apple. It is what you will eat that counts.

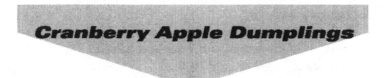

Cranberry Apple Dumplings

A high soluble fiber and high monounsaturated fat recipe

A FRESH CUT apple a day is still the best way to consume an apple. Another delicious apple is a baked apple. Here is a baked apple for special occasions.

This pie crust is easily made. It can be mixed with a fork. Flour, canola oil, and skim milk are the only ingredients. If you wish to peel the apple, the total fiber is then less, but still a healthful 2.7 grams, and the soluble fiber is 1 gram. Top your warm dumpling with milk, a sprinkling of cinnamon and oat bran, and serve.

1⅓ cup	unbleached flour
⅓ cup	canola or olive oil
3 tbs.	skim milk
8 small	Red Delicious apples, cored
3 tbs.	cranberries
3 tbs.	chopped pecans
8 tsp.	brown sugar
	Cinnamon (optional)
	Oat bran (optional)

1. Combine the flour, oil, and milk in a bowl. Press into two balls. Flatten one ball slightly and roll it between waxed paper to about an 8-inch round. Peel off the top paper. Cut the pie crust into 4 parts. Take one part and place an apple into the center of the crust. Fill the cored apple center with some cranberries, chopped pecans, and a teaspoon of brown sugar. Pull the dough over the apple and press around the apple. Some milk can be brushed over the crust to aid browning. Continue with the remaining dough and apples.
2. Place the dough-covered apples on a greased baking pan or baking sheet. Bake at 400° F for 20 minutes or until the apple is soft and the crust is golden. Let cool a bit but serve warm.

{ Yield: 8 servings }

Per serving: 269 calories, 3 g protein, 41 g carbohydrates, 12 g fat, 1 g sat fat, 7 g mono fat, 3 g poly fat, 1 mg cholesterol, 5 g dietary fiber, 1.5 g soluble fiber, 5 mg sodium.

More Quick Ways to Add Fiber

Remember: *there is no fiber in animal products.* Fiber, both soluble and insoluble, is found only in plants. So that means that meat, poultry, fish, milk, cheese, and eggs do not contain *any* fiber. Add at least two servings, or better yet three, of fruits and vegetables to each meal.

What's the Best Bread?

If you are reading the label on a package of bread, the first ingredient should be whole wheat or 100 percent whole wheat. If you want to make sure that it is whole wheat flour or contains other whole grains—not just wheat flour, which often means just white flour—you can tell by checking the fiber content. It should have at least 3 grams of fiber per 1-ounce slice. Fiber controls your appetite because it makes you feel full. You won't eat as much. Fiber also helps to lower cholesterol and keep you regular.

To get the fiber you need:

For breakfast. Top a bowl of whole-grain or fiber-rich hot or cold cereal with fruit, dried fruit, or nuts for additional fiber.

High-fiber snacks. When you need a quick energy boost during the day, reach for a high-fiber treat. Popcorn, fresh fruit, dried fruit, raw vegetables, or nuts are convenient and healthful choices.

"Fiberize." Substitute higher-fiber ingredients in recipes. Swap up to one-third of the flour with quick or old-fashioned oats when you bake. Add extra vegetables to casseroles, soups, salads, and pasta dishes. Use brown rice instead of white rice.

White or Brown Rice?

Should you choose white or brown rice? Is brown rice really healthier? Brown rice is the least processed rice; it is the whole grain, so it still contains the bran layer. The bran holds some of the vitamins and minerals in it, and this includes vitamin E. The bran also contains insoluble fiber. The dietary fiber, the rice bran oil, and a substance in the bran called oryzanol help to reduce the body's production of cholesterol.

The disadvantage to brown rice in these days of "quick" meals is that regular brown rice takes about 40 to 45 minutes to cook. But there is also a quick brown rice. Converted rice, both white and brown, retains more of the original nutrients after processing.

Try quick or converted brown rice or a combination of brown and white in this recipe that contains antioxidants, monounsaturated fats, and soluble fiber. Notice that using two whole eggs in a recipe that serves six means that each person gets about a third of an egg, and that doesn't make much difference in the amount of total daily cholesterol or saturated fat. You do have the choice of using egg substitutes.

Chicken Fried Rice

A brown rice recipe high in monounsaturated fat

2 tbs.	canola or olive oil
¼ cup	chopped mushrooms
¼ cup	chopped onion
½ cup	chopped sweet red pepper
¼ cup	chopped celery
3 cups	cooked brown or white rice, or a combination
½ cup	cooked green peas (or thawed frozen peas)
½ cup	diced cooked chicken
2	eggs, slightly beaten, or Egg Beaters™
2 tbs.	chopped unsalted, roasted cashews
	Low-sodium soy sauce or tamari (optional)
	Rice noodles (optional)

1. Heat the oil in a sauté pan. Add the mushrooms, onion, red pepper, and celery. Sauté until the vegetables are tender.
2. Remove the vegetables to a dish and set aside. Add the rice to the pan and sauté just to heat. Add the vegetables, peas, chicken, and slightly beaten eggs or Egg Beaters™.
3. Stir fry for 2 to 3 minutes, just until the chicken is heated and the egg is set. Place in a serving dish. Top with chopped cashews. Serve with soy sauce and rice noodles if desired. (Rice noodles have a little less fat in them than the traditional canned or packaged Chinese noodles used as a topping.)

❴ **Yield: 6 servings** ❵

Per serving: 194 calories, 9 g protein, 20 g carbohydrates, 2 g dietary fiber, 0.5 g soluble fiber, 9 g fat, 5 g mono fat, 2 g poly fat, 2 g sat fat, 81 mg cholesterol, 40 mg sodium. High in vitamin C, selenium, and vitamin A.

Bagels: The Other White Bread

Many clients tell me they had a bagel for breakfast, as if I would reply, "That's great!" Unfortunately, like white bread, bagels are devoid of fiber, unless you like sesame or poppy seeds on top. And bagels are getting bigger and bigger. They are getting to be so big that they are equal in calories to eating four slices of bread. So watch those portions. The original Lender's bagel is about 2.85 ounces, almost 3 servings, and 220 calories, 2 g of fat, and 430 mg of sodium. Some of the larger bagels are 4 ounces, or four servings; so eat just half a bagel and add some fiber to it. Chunky peanut butter, for example, would add some fiber and some monounsaturated fat. A bagel every day for breakfast is not the best use of your calories.

Think of other ways you can add fiber to your favorite recipes.

Learn About Phytochemicals and Antioxidants

Change No. 2. Enjoy foods rich in phytochemicals and the antioxidant vitamins: vitamin C, found in strawberries and citrus fruits; vitamin E, found in seeds, nuts, fortified ready-to-eat cereals, and whole grains; beta-carotene, found in dark green and yellow vegetables and fruits.

Antioxidants are necessary to prevent the oxidation or destruction of unsaturated fatty acids in the cells. When the destruction occurs, substances called **free radicals** are produced. These can damage healthy cells. Antioxidants prevent the free radicals from doing damage, causing the cholesterol to stick to the arteries, for example. The vitamin E in oils helps prevent the oils from getting rancid (being oxidized).

Phytochemicals are plant chemicals that scientists believe can prevent disease and maintain a healthy immune system. We know that unprocessed foods contain vitamins and minerals, and we are just beginning to know about other beneficial nutrients that are found in foods. For example, there is a phytochemical in the flavonoid category called *quercetin* that is found in tea, wine, apples, onions, and celery. Quercetin is one of the phytochemicals that help prevent heart disease.

When you are planning your menus and making judgments about foods, make sure phytochemicals are included. All the phytochemicals are found in plants: fruits, vegetables, whole grains, and nuts.

An aspirin a day has been suggested to help prevent heart disease. Aspirin is a salicylate, and a recent study found that salicylates are found in varied degrees in many vegetables and fruits. Vegetables high in salicylates include broccoli, chili peppers, cucumber, okra, spinach, squash, sweet potato, canned tomatoes, tomato paste and sauce, green peppers, radishes, and zucchini.

Herbs and spices high in salicylates include cayenne, celery powder, cinnamon, curry, dill, fenugreek, mustard, oregano, paprika, rosemary, sage, tarragon, turmeric, thyme, mint, black pepper, bay leaves, basil, caraway, ginger, and nutmeg.

Gouda and Strawberry Salad

A main dish salad, high in monounsaturated fat, folate, and soluble fiber

THIS DELICIOUS AND attractive salad can be a main dish, especially since it contains 300 calories and 12 g of protein. It is high in fat, although most of the fat comes from the pecans and the olive oil, which are high in the good monounsaturated oils. The cheese contributes 308

mg of calcium, which is important for bone health and keeping the blood pressure down. Use smaller amounts of the nuts, cheese, and dressing if you want to cut some fat. The recipe is high in monounsaturated fat, vitamin A, vitamin C, folate, and calcium.

8 cups	romaine, spinach, or radicchio greens
6 oz.	Gouda cheese, cut into bite-size slices
1½ cups	sliced juicy red strawberries
½ cup	toasted ground pecans
	Strawberry vinaigrette (recipe below)

1. The greens, cheese, and strawberries can be placed in a bowl and topped with the toasted ground pecans. Or place the greens on four salad plates. Arrange the cheese and strawberries on the greens. Divide the dressing between the four plates and garnish with 2 tablespoons of toasted ground pecans.

To Make the Strawberry Vinaigrette:
  2 tbs. seedless strawberry jam or strawberry preserves
  4 tbs. extra virgin olive oil
  4 tbs. red wine vinegar
  Salt and pepper to taste (optional)

2. Whisk all the ingredients together in a small bowl. Place in a jar with a lid until ready to use.

〔 **Yield: 6 servings** 〕

Per serving: 277 calories, 9 g protein, 12 g carbohydrates, 3 g dietary fiber, 22 g fat, 7 g sat fat, 12 g mono fat, 32 mg cholesterol, 240 mg sodium. Recipe adapted from the American Dairy Association web site, *www.ilovecheese.com.*

Pay Attention to Fat and Cholesterol Content

Change No. 3. Choose foods low in saturated fat, total fat, trans fat, and cholesterol by selecting lean meats and low-fat or nonfat dairy foods.

Reducing your cholesterol intake does lower your risk of heart disease, but it has less impact on blood cholesterol levels than cutting back on saturated fat and trans fat.

Saturated fat boosts your blood cholesterol level more than anything else in your diet. Eating less saturated fat is the best way to lower your cholesterol level. Saturated fat is found mainly in food that comes from animals. Whole-milk dairy products such as butter, cheese, milk, cream, and ice cream all contain high amounts of saturated fat. The fat in meat and poultry skin is loaded with saturated fat. A few vegetable fats—coconut oil, cocoa butter, palm kernel oil, and palm oil—are also high in saturated fat. These fats may be found in cookies, crackers, coffee creamers, whipped toppings, and snack foods. Because fats are invisible in many foods, it is important to read food labels, which detail total fat and saturated fat levels.

Several years ago French fries were commonly fried in beef fat. Removing animal fats to lower the saturated fat became important, so the fast-food restaurants and cookie and cracker manufacturers substituted vegetable oils. Unfortunately, many vegetable oils become rancid easily, especially at high temperatures, so the oils are hydrogenated to make them more stable. This also produces trans fats. Now people are asking, "Did we simply substitute one blood vessel clogger for another?"

Eat Foods Low in Saturated Fat and Cholesterol

Instead of	*Try*
High-fat meats	Lean meats, poultry without skin, fish
Bacon	Turkey bacon, lean ham, Canadian Bacon
Pork or beef sausage	Turkey or chicken sausage
Whole milk	1% or skim
Whole-milk cheeses	Low-fat or part-skim milk cheeses
Cream, evaporated milk	Evaporated skim milk
Sour cream	Low-fat or fat-free sour cream
Yogurt	Fat-free or low-fat yogurt
Lard, butter, shortening	Olive oil or canola oil
Regular mayonnaise	Mustard and nonfat or low-fat mayonnaise
Regular salad dressing	Low-fat or nonfat salad dressing; olive oil and vinegar dressings

Let's Talk About Cookies for a Minute

The following table shows the amount of various fats in different types of cookies:

Cookie	Calories	Total Fat	Sat Fat	Mono Fat	Trans Fat	Cholesterol
1 Vienna Finger	75 cal	3 g	0.75 g	?	?	0
1 Vienna Finger (reduced fat)	70	2.25 g	0.5 g	1 g	0.75 g	0
1 regular Oreo	53 cal	2.33 g	0.5 g	?	?	0
1 Oreo, (reduced fat)	47 ca	1.16 g	33	0.33 g	0.5 g	0
1 Double Stuff Oreo	70 cal	3.5 g	0.75	?	?	0
1 Newman-O	65 cal	2.25 g	0.75	?	0	0

Notice that all the cookies have zero cholesterol, and they do all contain fat. The amounts shown are for one cookie, but who can eat just one? Once you eat two, only the reduced-fat cookies are low in fat. The oil used in the Newman-O is organic palm oil, so labels can say "no trans fat and no cholesterol and lower in saturated fat than butter." These claims are all true, but notice the comparison with the other cookies. It's really not much different. The Newman-O package says, "Of the three tropical oils, palm oil is 50 percent saturated, palm kernel oil is 86 percent and coconut oil is 92 percent." (See the table in Chapter 1 for saturated fat comparisons.) Butter, beef fat, and palm oil are very similar in saturated fat content.

It is the total fat and saturated fat that causes the problem. It is the extra calories that cause triglycerides to go up. All you need is 100 extra calories a day to gain 10 pounds a year, and your body doesn't care where the calories come from to gain weight. Your heart cares though, if those extra calories are coming from saturated fat or trans fat.

Quick Vegetable Soup

A low-fat, low-saturated fat, and low-cholesterol recipe

I LOVE SOUPS, but often don't want to take the time to prepare them. Most canned soups are so high in sodium that I don't want to use them. This soup can be prepared easily and quickly and is low in sodium. Using homemade chicken broth will keep the sodium low.

This soup is a good way to use leftover cooked vegetables. Make sure they are low sodium if canned or no salt added if frozen.

2 cups	low-sodium vegetable juice
1 cup	low-fat and low-sodium chicken broth
2 cups	vegetables: carrots, mushrooms, green beans, green pepper, corn
½ cup	chopped onion
1	apple, peeled and cubed
½ cup	cubed, cooked chicken (no skin)
½ tsp.	curry powder
1 cup	cooked noodles (or rice)
	Dash ground black pepper

Combine the vegetable juice, broth, vegetables, onion, apple, soy and curry in a saucepan. Bring to a boil; lower heat, cover, and cook until the vegetables are tender, about 5 to 10 minutes. Add the noodles and black pepper and heat through.

〔 **Yield: 4 cups** 〕

Per cup: 179 calories, 11 g protein, 29 g carbohydrates, 5 g dietary fiber, 2 g soluble fiber, 2 fat, 0.5 g sat fat, 29 mg cholesterol, 158 mg sodium.

The Food Pyramid

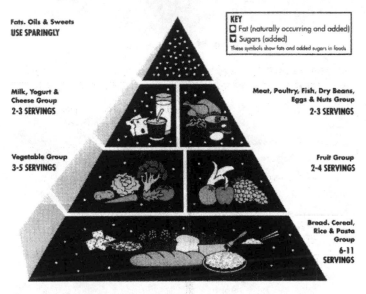

Fats. Oils & Sweets
USE SPARINGLY

KEY
☐ Fat (naturally occurring and added)
☑ Sugars (added)
These symbols show fats and added sugars in foods

Milk, Yogurt &
Cheese Group
2-3 SERVINGS

Meat, Poultry, Fish, Dry Beans,
Eggs & Nuts Group
2-3 SERVINGS

Vegetable Group
3-5 SERVINGS

Fruit Group
2-4 SERVINGS

Bread, Cereal,
Rice & Pasta
Group
6-11
SERVINGS

Source: United States Department of Agriculture

Following the Food Pyramid of the U.S. Department of Agriculture is a good basis for getting your dietary cholesterol under control. Each day, aim to include selections from the following food groups:

- Breads, cereals, rice, and pasta: 6 to 11 servings
- Vegetables: 3 to 5 servings
- Fruits: 2 to 4 servings
- Milk, yogurt, and cheese: 2 to 3 servings
- Meat, poultry, fish, dry beans and peas, eggs, nuts, and seeds: 2 to 3 servings
- (Use fats, oils, and sweets sparingly.)

Serving Size

Be careful about what you call a serving. The government recommendations aren't the same as the serving size indicated on a package label. For example, a serving from the grain group, as defined by the U.S. Department of Agriculture, may include one slice of bread, while the serving listed on the package could be two slices. Below are serving sizes for major foods, to be used in interpreting the Food Pyramid recommendations:

Grain products group (bread, cereal, rice, and pasta):
- 1 slice bread
- 1 oz. ready-to-eat cereal
- 1/2 cup cooked cereal, rice, or pasta

Vegetable group:
- 1 cup raw leafy vegetables
- 1/2 cup other vegetables—cooked or chopped raw
- 3/4 cup vegetable juice

Fruit group:
- 1 medium apple, banana, or orange
- 1/2 cup chopped, cooked, or canned fruit
- 3/4 cup fruit juice

Milk group (milk, yogurt, and cheese):
- 1 cup of milk or yogurt
- 1 1/2 oz. of natural cheese
- 2 oz. of processed cheese

Meat and beans group (meat, poultry, fish, dry beans, eggs, and nuts):
- 2–3 oz. of cooked lean meat, poultry, or fish
- 1/2 cup of cooked dry beans or 1 egg counts as 1 oz. lean meat. Two tbs. peanut butter or 1/3 cup nuts count as 1 oz. meat.

Specific Dietary Suggestions
for Reducing Blood Cholesterol Levels

▶ Lean toward fruits, vegetables, and whole grains for the basis of your meals.

▶ Limit meat to 5 to 6 ounces of fish, poultry, or lean cuts per day. Remove fat and skin before eating. Avoid processed meats, such as sausage, bacon, and high-fat cold cuts. Avoid organ meats, such as liver, kidney, or brains.

▶ Drink skim or 1 percent milk instead of whole milk. Switch to low-fat or nonfat cheeses and yogurt.

▶ Avoid fried foods in favor of broiled, baked, roasted, or poached alternatives.

▶ Concentrate on cutting back fat from all sources, and you will be cutting down on saturated fat, too. Use healthier fats in place of saturated fats, as described below.

▶ Substitute olive oil for butter. If you use about a teaspoon of butter on a slice of bread now, you could substitute a teaspoon of olive oil and get more of the monounsaturated fat than the saturated fat in the butter. (If you eat a lot of bread and add a tablespoon of spread to each slice, you are eating too much fat. You might be a candidate for Benecol or Take Control, mentioned in Chapter 6.)

▶ Add the omega-3 fatty acids, which are found in fish and also in soybean and canola oils. Add fish to your diet once or twice a week, and choose soy and canola oils. The jury is still out on whether fish oil supplements are beneficial over the long term. It is always better to eat the fish.

▶ Add soy: You may have heard about the cholesterol-cutting benefits of soy protein. The Food and Drug Administration recently said that soy protein in a diet low in saturated fat and cholesterol may help reduce the risk of heart disease. Soy protein can be found in many products, including soy milk, tofu, tempeh, soy-based meat alternatives, soy nuts, soy butter, and even soy yogurt. Bear in mind, though, that it takes 25 grams of soy protein daily to produce a significant cholesterol-lowering effect. That's about 3½ cups of soy milk or more than 10 ounces of tofu daily.

Here's the key take-home message: Heart disease has a clear connection with fat intake. To lose weight and to lower your total and LDL cholesterol, be sure to stick with a program that keeps total fat to no more than 30 percent of your daily calories, with saturated fat constituting no more than 10 percent. Use the menus in Chapter 10 that are low in fat, cholesterol, and saturated fat as a guide.

9

FOODS THAT MAKE THE DIFFERENCE: HOW TO MODIFY RECIPES TO MAKE THEM HEALTHIER

To improve your cholesterol levels, it is important not only to remember the foods you have to omit from your diet, but also the foods you need to add. Foods you can add, for example, are the high-fiber foods, especially those high in soluble fiber, such as oats and oat bran, garlic, beans, and carrots. The fatty ocean fish with high levels of omega-3 fatty acids have been mentioned several times as helping to keep your arteries open.

Foods and Fiber

The Journal of the American Medical Association reports that a diet high in fiber may help control weight and reduce the risk of heart disease. In a study of 2,900 adults who were tracked over a period of 10 years, it was found that the people who consumed the most dietary fiber were more likely to be at a healthy weight and also to have better insulin control. Good insulin control means you're less likely to get the disease known as diabetes. A diet high in soluble fiber provides some protection from heart disease by preventing cholesterol absorption from the intestine.

The American Dietetic Association recommends that 20–35 grams of dietary fiber be included in the diet every day. Look in Chapter 10 for menus that will show how this much fiber can easily be included daily.

Foods That Are High in Soluble Fiber

Foods that are highest in soluble fiber and total dietary fiber are fruits, vegetables, legumes, and grains. It is best to aim for 6–10 servings of these foods every day. Here is a list of some foods that are high in soluble fiber and total fiber.

Food	Amount	Soluble Fiber (grams)	Total fiber (grams)
Brussels sprouts	1 cup	2.6	5
Kidney beans (cooked)	½ cup	2.8	6.9
Navy beans (cooked)	½ cup	2.2	6.5
Figs, dried	3	2.2	4.6
Oat bran	⅓ cup	2	4
Orange	1	1.8	2.9
Baked potato	1	1.2	5
Baked sweet potato	1	1.2	2.7
Blackberries	¾ cup	1.1	3.7
Carrot	1	1.1	2.3
Pear	1 small	1.1	2.9
Apple with skin	1 small	1	2.8
Barley (raw)	2 tbs.	0.9	3
Wheat germ (toasted)	¼ cup	0.8	5.2

The DASH Diet

Including six to ten servings of high-fiber foods is not only good for lowering cholesterol, it is advised for lowering blood pressure as well. The DASH (Dietary Approaches to Stop Hypertension) diet is an eating plan that has been proven to lower blood pressure and also helps bring down blood cholesterol.

There is only one healthy way to eat. There is not one healthy diet to prevent osteoporosis, one to lower LDL cholesterol, and another to keep your blood pressure low. If you follow the DASH diet, you will simultaneously lower your blood pressure and your LDL (Low Down Lousy) cholesterol, and hence your risk for heart disease.

The DASH diet includes:

- **Fruits and vegetables**: 10 servings a day
- **Low-fat or nonfat dairy foods**: The calcium in these foods helps to lower blood pressure. The big three minerals—potassium, magnesium, and calcium— together help to lower blood pressure. Potassium and magnesium are in fruits, vegetables, and whole grains.
- **Low fat**: All the other information about a healthy diet that you have heard applies to the DASH diet as well: keep fat, especially saturated and trans fat, low, and cut down on red meat.
- **Low sugar**: The DASH diet is also low in sweets and sugar-containing drinks.
- **Low sodium**: Last, and most important, is to keep your salt intake low, as low as possible. I still hear that lowering salt intake only applies to those who are susceptible to high blood pressure. This is *wrong;* it applies to everyone. All those in the study—old and young, men and women, black and white, fat and thin, active and not—were affected by salt intake: Their blood pressure went down. The lower the salt intake, the more the blood pressure went down. (Note: To those who already have low blood pressure, follow the advice of your doctor concerning the amount of salt to consume.)

Modifying Recipes From Original to Healthier to Healthiest

Do you have favorite family recipes that use a lot of fat? Are you afraid that embarking on a new low-fat lifestyle will mean you won't be able to serve these family favorites anymore?

Don't despair. Recipes can be modified to make them healthier. You can take recipes that you use regularly and modify them to help you lower your cholesterol.

Many cooks fear that they won't like their own recipes if they are prepared in a healthier way. They think that oat bran, plain yogurt, and fat-free products are what they have to eat from now on—in other words, that they have to give up good-tasting food. This isn't true.

Where should you start? I'm going to show you how to modify your old favorites in a two-step process, first showing how to make them healthier, and then how to make them healthiest. Following are some modifications you will want to make:

Cut out or use fewer high-fat items. What you have to do is to move from whole milk to low-fat milk to skim milk. Or you might stop at the second step, the low-fat milk, which is a step in the right direction. You can stop there if you lose weight, your blood pressure goes down, you have more energy, or your cholesterol drops. If you find some benefits to a healthy diet, you may continue onward to step 2.

The first-step recipes are healthier because they are lower in fat. They contain close to 30 percent of their calories from fat, which is what you are aiming for if you want to reduce your LDL cholesterol levels. The second-step recipes result in foods that have 20 percent of their calories from fat.

Cut out or use fewer high-salt items. Recipes and foods should be low in sodium. Read labels, and find foods that have less than 300 mg per serving of sodium.

Add more high-fiber items. Think high fiber and add vegetables, grains, and fruits to your recipes so they will contain more dietary fiber. You might be eating white rice now. Can you give brown rice a chance? Or a quick brown rice? Combine quick brown and white?

There are many whole grains you can add to your diet for more nutrients and fiber: quick barley, bulgur, quick oats, millet, wild rice, quinoa, spelt, and teff. Try a new whole grain. Use it in soups and salads. Choose barley and mushroom soup in a restaurant rather than the high-fat onion soup.

Healthier Macaroni and Cheese

From a Boxed Mix

Instead of preparing the recipe exactly according to the directions on the box, be inventive.

Step 1:

Use half the butter or half the margarine called for in the directions.

Use a lower-fat milk.

Use only half the powdered cheese mix to cut down on sodium.

Add more macaroni *or* a whole-wheat macaroni, which adds fiber and also gives you more servings. This means each serving will have less fat and sodium.

Step 2:

Use skim milk as the liquid of choice. Use even less fat or switch to a monounsaturated oil like canola or olive oil instead of using margarine or butter. Add fiber—chopped onion, tomato, and garlic. Add 1 cup of snow peas, a package of frozen peas and carrots, or stewed tomatoes. A drained can of tuna adds omega-3 fatty acids. I hope I have you thinking creatively!

From a Recipe

Original Macaroni and Cheese

High fat, high saturated fat, high salt, and little fiber

1½ cups	uncooked elbow macaroni
2	eggs
1 cup	milk
¼ tsp.	red pepper
⅛ tsp.	black pepper
½ tsp.	salt
3 cups	shredded Cheddar cheese

1. To prepare the macaroni, bring a quart of water to a boil. Add the macaroni and cook over medium-high heat for 10 minutes. Drain, and stop the cooking by rinsing with cold water.
2. While the elbows are cooking, beat the eggs in a small bowl. Whisk in the milk and dried red and black pepper.
3. Spoon one-third of the cooked macaroni into a greased 9 x 13 baking dish. Cover with one cup of the cheese, then another third of the elbows, and then another cup of cheese, and then the remaining elbows, and finally the last cup of cheese. Then pour the egg mixture over it all.
4. Cover with foil and bake at 350°F for 45 to 60 minutes.

❨ **Yield: 4–6 servings.** ❩

Per serving: 558 calories, 31 g protein, 33 g carbohydrate, 33 g fat, 54 percent calories from fat, 20 g sat fat, 879 mg sodium, 1.36 g dietary fiber, 0.2 g soluble fiber, and 203 mg cholesterol.

〉 Step 1: *Healthier Macaroni and Cheese*

LOWER-FAT MILK and cheese are substituted for the full-fat products. More macaroni is added. Egg substitutes are used instead of eggs to cut down on cholesterol and fat. Hot pepper flakes are added for flavor since low-fat cheese products are usually bland.

2 cups	uncooked elbow macaroni
½ cup	egg substitute or one egg and two whites
1 cup	reduced-fat or 2-percent milk
¼ tsp.	dried red pepper flakes
⅛ tsp.	black pepper
3 cups	low-fat shredded cheddar

1. Cook the macaroni in 1½ quarts boiling water for 10 minutes or until tender. Drain and rinse with cold water.
2. Beat the egg substitute in a bowl. Beat in the skim milk and the red and black pepper.
3. Spray a 9 x 13 pan with nonstick spray. Add one third of the cooked elbows to the pan. Cover the elbows with a cup of the cheese. Add another third of the elbows and cover with another cup of cheese. Add the remaining elbows and cover with the remaining cheese. Now pour the milk mixture over all of it.
4. Cover and bake at 350°F for 40 to 60 minutes.

〈 Yield: 4–6 servings 〉

Per serving: 296 calories, 18g protein, 42 g carbohydrates, 6 g fat (18 percent calories from fat), 4 g sat fat, 539 mg sodium, and 2 gm dietary fiber, 0.27g soluble fiber, 20mg cholesterol.

❯ Step 2: *Healthiest Macaroni and Cheese*

MORE HERBS ARE added for flavor because the salt is omitted. Vegetables are added for fiber and soluble fiber. Skim milk or evaporated skim milk is substituted for the reduced-fat milk. Because more ingredients are added, the servings are now larger, but there are only 70 more calories per serving than the healthier recipe, with more healthy fiber.

2 cups	elbow macaroni
½ cup	egg substitute or 2 egg whites
1 cup	skim milk or evaporated skim milk
1 teaspoon	dried onion flakes
½ tsp.	garlic powder
¼ tsp.	red pepper flakes (or your favorite hot pepper sauce, to taste)
⅛ tsp.	black pepper
10 oz.	frozen peas and carrots, thawed and drained
14 oz. can	no-salt-added stewed tomatoes
3 cups	reduced-fat cheddar, shredded
2 tbs.	grated parmesan
2 tbs.	minced fresh parsley

1. Cook macaroni. Drain.
2. Combine the egg substitute, skim milk, onion, garlic powder, red pepper flakes, black pepper, peas and carrots, tomatoes, reduced-fat cheddar, and cooked macaroni. Pour into a 9 x 13 inch, nonstick, sprayed baking dish. Cover with the parmesan cheese that has been mixed with the parsley.
3. Bake uncovered at 400°F for 20 minutes, or until golden on top.

❮ **Yield: 4–6 servings** ❯

Per serving: 366 calories, 23g protein, 55 g carbohydrates, 6 g fat (15 percent calories from fat), 3.5 g sat fat, 370 mg sodium, 5.8 g dietary fiber, 0.85 g soluble fiber, 19 mg cholesterol.

Original Chili

A CHILI RECIPE from the 1960s or '70s would take two hours to prepare and then would provide large portions. Recipes in those days would say "Skim if necessary," meaning to take off the top layer of fat. Of course, not too many did that; they enjoyed the taste of the fat.

    4 tbs. fat or Crisco
    1 cup thinly sliced onions
    2 lbs. ground chuck
    2-3 tbs. chili powder
    1½ cups boiling water
    2½ cups canned tomatoes
    1 tsp. salt
    2 tsp. sugar
    1 tsp. dehydrated minced garlic
    2 cups canned or cooked kidney beans

Melt the fat in a skillet and brown the meat in it. Then add the remaining ingredients, except for the beans and cook—covered, for an hour and then uncovered for ½ hour. Add the beans and heat through.

❰ Yield: 6 servings ❱

Per serving: 534 calories, 34 g protein, 21 g carbohydrates, 35 g fat, (59 percent calories from fat), 14 g sat fat, 17 g mono fat, 104 mg cholesterol, 924 mg sodium, 5 g dietary fiber, 1 g soluble fiber.

❯ *Step 1: **Healthier Chili***

TO BROWN THE meat, less fat is used. Olive oil is substituted for the shortening. Lean meat is used, and less of it. The amount of beans is doubled and the salt and sugar are omitted.

2 tbs.	olive oil
3	small cloves garlic, minced
1 cup	thinly sliced onions
1 lb.	extra lean ground beef
2 tbs.	chili powder
1½	cups water
2½	cups canned tomatoes, no salt added
2 (15 oz.) cans	kidney beans

Heat the oil in a pot. Add the garlic, onions, and beef and cook until the beef is browned and the onions have softened. Then add the chili powder, water, tomatoes, and sugar, and cook, covered, for 30 minutes, then uncover for 30 minutes. Add the beans and heat through.

❮ Yield: 6 servings ❯

Per serving: 325 calories, 25 g protein, 30 g carbohydrates, 12 g fat, 34 percent calories from fat, 4 g sat fat, 6 g mono fat, 28 mg cholesterol, 737 mg sodium, 8 g dietary fiber, 1.7 g soluble fiber.

⟩ *Step 2:* **Healthiest Chili**

IN THE STEP 2 chili, ground turkey or chicken is substituted for the beef. Read the labels for the fat content or buy turkey breast and grind it yourself. That way, you know that skin and fat are not included in the mix.

More vegetables are added. You can substitute red beans or pinto beans for the kidney beans for variety. You can cook beans from scratch, or you can use beans canned without salt to avoid too much sodium. Serve the chili over brown rice for added fiber. The thickness of the liquid in the canned beans is the soluble fiber, so it is better to use salt-free canned beans because if you rinse the beans, you are throwing away some of the fiber.

2 tbs.	olive oil
1 cup	chopped onions
3	cloves garlic, minced
1 cup	chopped celery
1 lb.	ground turkey
1	carrot, shredded or finely chopped
½ cup	chopped green pepper
2 tbs.	chili powder
1 tsp.	ground cumin
½ tsp.	ground allspice
¼ tsp.	black pepper
2½ cups	canned tomatoes in puree
½ cup	water to rinse out can
¼ cup	red wine
6 cups	cooked kidney beans, no salt added

1. Heat the oil in a large (8 quart) pot. Add the onion, garlic, and celery, and sauté for 5 minutes. Add the turkey and cook for 10 minutes. Add the carrot, green pepper, chili powder, cumin, allspice, and pepper and combine well. Then add the tomatoes, the water to rinse out can, and the red wine. Cook for 20 minutes.

2. Add the beans and heat through. Serve on cooked rice. Pass the hot pepper sauce.

〔 Yield: 6–10 〕

Per serving: 413 calories, 36 g protein, 53 g carbohydrate, 6.6 g fat (14 percent calories from fat), 1 g sat fat, 47 mg cholesterol, 15 g dietary fiber, 5.6 g soluble fiber, 242 mg sodium.

How About Modifying a Cake?

Your favorite cake recipes can be modified to make them lower in fat, calories, saturated fat, cholesterol, and even sodium.

Try removing some of the fat in a recipe. For example, instead of using one stick of butter, use half a stick. And instead of using butter, use a margarine that contains mainly vegetable oil and no trans fatty acids. Promise margarine is one of the margarines that contains no trans fatty acids.

The amount of fat that you omit can be replaced with applesauce, any pureed fruit, or low-fat or nonfat yogurt or sour cream.

The amount of sugar in a recipe can be cut somewhat to lower the total calories. If you remove a small amount, for example, a quarter cup of sugar, you will not notice the difference in the final product, and the calories will be lowered slightly.

Baking powder and baking soda contain sodium. If these products are in a recipe, the salt in the recipe can be omitted to lower the sodium content.

By making little changes every time you prepare a recipe, you can get a healthier recipe that will still taste good.

Orange Pound Cake

THE ORIGINAL POUND cake recipe contained $3/4$ cup of half-and-half and one stick of butter. Nonfat plain yogurt was substituted for the half-and-half. Instead of using one stick of butter, $1/2$ a stick of margarine and $1/4$ cup of plain nonfat yogurt were substituted. Originally there was $3/4$ cup of whole milk yogurt in the cake.

To lower the fat even more, some of the whole eggs could be omitted. Because I didn't want to change the texture too much from the original, I did not make that change. Often one or two substitutions can be made without noticing a big change in the texture or taste.

The result is still a tasty pound cake. Make sure you only eat one portion, or even half a portion, to satisfy your sweet tooth. In each serving there are 5 grams of fat, which is much lower than the 11 grams of the original. There is only 1.4 grams of saturated fat compared with the original recipe's 6.3 grams, which was higher than the total amount of fat in the cake as it is now. The cholesterol content is 71 mg, which could be lowered with the use of egg substitutes or egg whites substituted for some or all of the eggs. Those eggs in the ingredients are divided into 12 portions.

4	eggs
1¼	cup sugar
1/2 tsp.	salt
1 cup	plain nonfat yogurt
1 tbs.	grated or chopped orange peel
1¾ cup	unbleached flour
1 ¼ tsp.	baking powder
¼ cup	margarine, melted and cooled or olive oil
¼ cup	orange juice

1. Preheat the oven to 325° F degrees. Spray a 9 x 5 inch loaf pan with a nonstick spray.
2. Beat the eggs with an electric mixer. Slowly add the sugar and salt and beat until fluffy. Beat in the yogurt and the orange peel.
3. Sift the flour with the baking powder. Add to the egg mixture and beat until smooth. Stir in the melted margarine. Pour the batter into the loaf pan and bake for $1^1/4$ hours. Cool the loaf in the pan.
4. Pierce the top of the cake with a toothpick and then pour the orange juice over the top of the cooled cake. Cool completely and then invert to remove.

❧ Yield: 12 slices ❧

Per slice: 221 calories (original 267 calories), 5 g fat (original 11 grams of fat), 1.4 g saturated fat (original 6.3 g), 71 mg cholesterol (original 99 mg), 206 mg sodium (original 255 mg sodium) 38 g carbohydrate, 6 g protein.

Start on Your Recipes Next

Now try modifying some of your own family favorite recipes in small steps. Each time you make the recipe, try to think of a good way to make it even healthier than before—without ruining the taste.

But don't stop with your old recipes. Seek new ones, and seek new food choices. Be creative. You'll be trying new foods and eating more of a varied and interesting diet than you ever thought possible. And you may even enjoy some of the foods that you had been laughing to your friends about. "Me eat cooked kale?" You'll have a healthier pantry. There will be new foods in your kitchen. You'll find you will be feeling better.

Don't panic. Take your time to make changes. After you use up the corn oil, switch to olive oil. As you use up your bottled salad dressings, make your own or just use olive oil and vinegar. If you have already cut back on meat and stopped eating fried foods, good for you. Maybe you have already cut back on eggs and stopped buying deli meats. Are you choosing low-fat dairy products? Are you being more discriminating in your choice of restaurants and fast-food spots? Can you omit commercial baked goods, cookies, and crackers—along with eating more fresh fruits and vegetables and whole-grain breads and cereals? Give yourself a pat on the back every time you do something good for yourself and your diet.

You, like almost everyone today, are interested in living longer—not just living more years but living a productive and healthy life. No one wants to be eighty years old and alive but crippled from a stroke, having to lead a sedentary life because of angina, sitting in the house attached to oxygen because of smoking-related emphysema, or sitting at home staring out the window for fear a fall might be fatal.

Of course there are those whose philosophy is "I will only live once and I'm going to enjoy it." They smoke and enjoy a doughnut every day. Don't be one of those people. Remember, it *is* what you do every day that counts.

10

MENUS THAT HELP TO LOWER TOTAL CHOLESTEROL AND LDL

Very few people who want to lower their cholesterol levels know what menus with 30 percent of the calories from fat look like. How different will your eating style have to be to get healthier and to reduce your risk of a heart attack or heart disease? In order to change, you need sample menus for at least a day.

Here is a week's worth of menus to help you lower your cholesterol. The menus incorporate the suggestions from Chapters 8 and 9. These are menus that require no specific recipes, so it should be easy for you to use them to eat in a healthy way without spending a great deal of time cooking. By following these patterns—and they are just patterns—you can see what 30 percent of the calories from fat could look like. Most of these menus include 20 percent of the calories from fat or even less. The idea that a percentage of calories from fat is a goal has no real practical value when eating. You just have to eat as little fat as you can, because there is so much hidden fat.

Several of the meals can also be eaten in restaurants. For example, there is an Asian meal that can be prepared at home or purchased in a restaurant. Many people like to eat out several times a week, and you can do that and still eat in a healthier way.

Not only will these menus help to lower your total cholesterol and your LDL, but they will also help prevent high blood pressure, because they follow the DASH diet and contain no more than 2,400 mg of sodium. They will help prevent osteo-porosis because they contain between 900 and 1,000 mg of cal-cium. These menus may also help prevent type 2 diabetes and obesity because they contain only 2,000 calories or less. That is what a healthy diet should do! However, note that everyone has slightly different calorie requirements. Men may need to add more calories, possibly bigger portions or servings. Women may need to eat less.

For example, a small woman might need only 1,300 calories to maintain her weight, so she would need to cut 600 to 700 calories from these menus. In Day 1, the beef in the Mexican lentil stew could be omitted (-50 calories), as well as the sour cream (-40 calories) and the pudding (-100 calories). A nonfat plain yogurt or skim milk, or another high-calcium food could be substituted (+50). The bread (-90) with the diet margarine (-33) could be omitted from dinner, and the pretzels (-220) could also be omitted. The vanilla ice milk (-100 calories) could be omitted and another high-calcium food substituted, such as ½ cup skim milk (+50).

A large man doing a lot of physical labor might need more than 2,000 calories a day. To increase the calories, it is best to add larger portions of vegetables or an extra slice of whole-wheat bread or another serving of a high-calcium food, such as the pudding or the ice milk.

Following are the recommendations of the National Cholesterol Education Program for a diet to reduce high cho-lesterol levels:

Step 1 Diet Guidelines

- Polyunsaturated fats: no more than 10 percent of daily calories
- Monounsaturated fats: no more than 15 percent of daily calories

- Saturated fats: no more than 10 per cent of daily calories
- Total fat: 30–35 percent of daily calories
- Carbohydrates: at least 55 percent
- Protein: approximately 15 percent
- Cholesterol: less than 300 mg per day
- Sodium: no more than 2,400 mg per day

If after three months on this diet your cholesterol is not reduced, then you will have to switch to the Step 2 Diet.

Step 2 Diet

The goals are the same as above, but the saturated fats are reduced to less than 7 percent of calories and the cholesterol is limited to 200 mg per day. The following menus incorporate the Step 1 guidelines, but most are lower in saturated fat and cholesterol and follow the Step 2 guidelines.

Day 1

Menu Tips

This menu recognizes that oatmeal is a good choice for breakfast. Oat bran is high in soluble fiber, which helps lower cholesterol, so a little extra is added on the cereal. Note that beef is used at both lunch and dinner; beef can be used as long as it is lean and as long as the portion size is close to 3 ounces. Ground turkey or chicken can be substituted for the lunch. If you are eating in a restaurant, an alternative to beef could be a vegetarian chili. Notice that even though beef is eaten twice during the day, the fat total is still low, only 16 percent of calories. It is much less than 30–35 percent, which is as high as you should go, according to the National Cholesterol Education Program guidelines.

Barley is used for dinner because that is a whole grain that is high in soluble fiber. The menu limits the use of sodium, since that is helpful in preventing high blood pressure, another risk for cardiovascular disease.

The menu contains at least seven servings of fruits and vegetables and six servings of grains. More fruits and vegetables can be added to help keep blood pressure low, but even with this amount of fruits, vegetables, and grains, there are 43 grams of dietary fiber in this menu, which is *very* high compared with the usual American diet. Men can have eleven servings of whole grains to add more calories.

If low- or reduced-fat dairy products are used, rather than skim, that will add more calories and fat.

Breakfast

〕 1 cup cooked oatmeal with 2 tsp. oat bran and ½ cup skim milk

〕 1 orange

Lunch

〕 Lentil Chili: 1 oz. extra-lean ground beef, ½ cup cooked lentils, 3 tbs. stewed tomatoes, ¼ chopped tomato, ½ cup chopped lettuce, 1 oz. shredded low-sodium, low-fat cheddar cheese, 2 tbs. mashed avocado, and 2 tbs. light sour cream

〕 1 cup steamed rice

〕 2 tbs. salsa, optional

〕 ½ cup vanilla pudding made with 2-percent or lower milk

Dinner

〕 Beef Stew: 2 oz. lean beef (bottom round), simmered in 1 cup water with ½ cup chunked carrots, 1 cup chunked potatoes, ½ cup sliced onions, 1 clove minced fresh garlic, 2 tbs. parsley, 1 tsp. basil and 1 tsp. savory

〕 ½ cup cooked barley or barley/rice mix, flavored with ¼ tsp. marjoram, 1 tbs. chopped onion, and ¼ tsp. garlic powder

〕 1 slice whole-wheat bread or low-sodium cornbread with 2 tsp. diet margarine

Snacks

〕 1 apple

〕 2 oz. unsalted pretzels

〕 ½ cup vanilla ice milk

> Daily totals: 1,901 calories, 31 g fat (14 percent of calories), 11 g saturated fat (5 percent of calories), 101 mg cholesterol, 40 g dietary fiber, 12 g soluble fiber, 1,072 mg sodium, 857 mg calcium, 320 g carbohydrates (67 percent of calories), 89 g protein (18 percent of calories).

Day 2

Menu Tips

Just remember it is what you do almost every day that counts. So if on a weekend you change a bit from your regular routine, well, that's OK. The American Heart Association recommends no more than seven egg yolks a week, so keep that in mind. If you eat oatmeal for breakfast every day and then have eggs on a weekend for breakfast, that's OK. If you enjoy going out for breakfast, many restaurants will make an omelette with just egg whites or with an egg substitute such as Egg Beaters.

Apples are high in soluble fiber, which is why you see them frequently in these menus. The lunch can be prepared at home or can be purchased at Wendy's. A baked potato with a broccoli and cheese topping and an individual salad can be ordered from the menu. Nuts make a good snack or a before-meal treat to take the edge off hunger. They add monounsaturated fats to the diet.

Breakfast

⟩ Scrambled eggs: ¼ cup egg substitute scrambled with 1 tbs. skim milk in a nonstick pan

⟩ 1 oz. turkey sausage

⟩ 1 toasted English muffin with 2 tbs. unsalted peanut butter and 2 tbs. strawberry jam

Lunch

⟩ Rice Jambalaya: 1½ cups cooked rice with 1/4 cup cooked diced ham, ¼ cup cooked cubed chicken breast, ¼ cup crushed no-salt tomatoes, ¼ cup diced celery, ¼ cup chopped onions, ¼ cup chopped green peppers, and ¼ cup chopped mushrooms

⟩ Fruit compote: 1 orange, sectioned, and 1 kiwifruit, sliced

Dinner

⟩ Stuffed potato: 1 baked potato with 1 oz. low-fat cheddar cheese, ½ cup steamed broccoli, ¼ cup chopped onions, and 1 clove fresh garlic, minced

⟩ 1 carrot, cut into sticks with 1 tbs. low-fat blue cheese dressing

⟩ ½ cup chocolate pudding, made with 2-percent (or lower) milk

Snacks

⟩ 1 stewed apple, topped with ¼ cup nonfat vanilla yogurt and drizzled with 1 tbs. of honey

⟩ 2 tbs. almonds

Daily totals: 1,960 calories, 44 g fat (19 percent of calories), 8.8 g saturated fat (4 percent of calories), 88 mg cholesterol, 31 g dietary fiber, 10 g soluble fiber, 1,779 mg sodium, 934 mg calcium, 322 g carbohydrate (64 percent of calories), 83 g protein (17 percent of calories).

Day 3

Menu Tips

What makes this menu special is the figs, which are high in soluble fiber; the abundance of vegetables, using only 3 ounces of grilled chicken breast; and two or more servings of fruit. The cookies are there for the person with a sweet tooth, but substituting fruit is better. Making your own cookies using an oil such as canola or peanut oil that is high in monounsaturated fat would also be a good thing. Commercial cookies are made with hydrogenated fats, which contain the bad trans fatty acids.

The yogurt and fruit for dessert at lunch can be saved to use as a nighttime snack. Lois Young, a high-cholesterol patient, likes to have fruited yogurt topped with grape nuts as an evening snack: it is sweet, low fat, and crunchy.

Remember to check labels for sodium content; with so much commercial food on this menu, you should choose the product that is the lowest in sodium. Commercial three-bean salad can be high in sodium. If the only brand you can find is high in sodium, make your own or substitute something lower in sodium. Beans are high in soluble fiber, but if they come with too much salt and you can't prepare your own, choose something else. Salad bars usually have a three-bean salad or chick peas. These menus point out that you can include more than 35 grams of dietary fiber in one day.

Breakfast

- 〗 ¾ cup orange juice
- 〗 1 cup ready-to-eat raisin bran cereal with ½ cup skim milk
- 〗 2 dried figs

Lunch

- 〗 Vegetable burger on whole-wheat bun with lettuce, tomato, onion, and mustard
- 〗 ½ cup commercially prepared three-bean salad
- 〗 1 carrot and 1 stalk celery, cut into sticks
- 〗 ½ cup low-fat, coffee-flavored yogurt
- 〗 1 tangerine or other fresh fruit

Dinner

- 〗 Tossed salad: 3 cups chopped romaine lettuce, 2 slices tomato, ½ sliced carrot, 2 radishes, 4 slices cucumber, dressed with 2 tsp. olive oil and 2 tbs. vinegar
- 〗 3 oz. grilled or baked chicken breast, rubbed with fresh garlic and ½ tsp. olive oil
- 〗 1 cup steamed brown rice
- 〗 ½ cup steamed Brussels sprouts
- 〗 1 baked apple with 2 tbs. maple syrup

Snacks

- 〗 2 fat-free cookies
- 〗 ½ cinnamon-raisin bagel with 1 tbs. low-fat cream cheese

> Daily totals: 1,852 calories, 34 g fat (16 percent of calories), 8.5 g saturated fat (4 percent of calories), 71 mg cholesterol, 39 g dietary fiber, 12g soluble fiber, 1,638 mg sodium, 1,022 mg calcium, 335 g carbohydrates (69 percent of calories), 73 g protein (15 percent of calories).

Day 4

Menu Tips

Fish is important, with its omega-3 fatty acid content, especially the fatty ocean fish, which have the highest omega-3 fatty acid content. Here, salmon is chosen for its healthful fat content.

Eat for the best or the most nutrition you can get for your calories. When you choose the food that has the most phytochemicals, vitamins, and minerals, then you are choosing the most nutrient-dense food.

To add more calories, add more turkey, another sandwich, some light mayonnaise spread, or more rice.

Breakfast

﹥ 1 slice toasted whole-wheat or five-grain bread with 2 tsp. diet margarine (trans fat-free) or a slice of fat-free cheese, melted

﹥ 1 cup low-fat vanilla yogurt with 2 chopped dried figs and 2 tsp. oat bran

Lunch

﹥ 1 cup grape juice

﹥ Roasted turkey breast sandwich with 1 oz. sliced turkey, lettuce, tomato, mustard, on whole-wheat bread

﹥ Spinach salad with 2 cups spinach, ½ carrot shredded, ¼ cup chickpeas, 2 tsp. olive oil, 2 tbs. cider vinegar

﹥ 4 graham crackers

Dinner

﹥ 4 oz. broiled salmon

﹥ 1 cups white and wild rice with 2 tsp. slivered almonds, 1

⟫ tbs. sautéed diced onions, 2 tsp. chopped parsley, and a
pinch of saffron

⟫ 1 artichoke, dressed with 1 tbs. lemon juice, 1 tsp. olive oil, 2
tsp parmesan cheese

⟫ ¼ wedge cantaloupe

Snack

⟫ Tropical shake: ½ cup skim milk, ½ cup orange juice, 1
banana, and 5 strawberries, whipped until thick and frothy

Daily totals: 1,908 calories, 51 g fat (23 percent of calories),
11 g saturated fat (5 percent of calories), 107 mg cholesterol, 33 g dietary fiber, ≥8 g soluble fiber, 1,755 mg sodium, 999 mg calcium, 300 g carbohydrates (60 percent of
calories), 83 g protein (17 percent of calories).

Day 5

Menu Tips

In this day's meals, lunch includes pizza, which is usually high
in sodium. If you go to a restaurant, it is difficult to know how
much salt is in the pizza, but when you get home if you have to
drink 2 to 3 glasses of water to quench your thirst, don't go back
to that place anymore.

Tomato sauces vary in their sodium content, as do cheeses.
Breads and pizza crusts are usually high in sodium, and if you
add any deli meats, such as pepperoni or sausage, they are high
in saturated fats and sodium, too. Ask for sliced fresh vegetables as toppings on pizza, or add some at home. They add fiber.
Extra oregano contributes more heart-healthy flavonoids.

The dietary fiber is high at 36 grams for the day. Remember,
fruit, vegetables, and grains are high in necessary fiber.

Breakfast

〗 1 cup oatmeal with ½ cup sliced strawberries, 1 tbs. brown sugar, and ½ cup skim milk

〗 1 slice toasted, whole-wheat bread with 1 oz. low-fat cheddar cheese

Lunch

〗 Pizza: ¼ of a pizza: ready-made pizza crust, ¼ cup tomato sauce, 1 oz. part-skim mozzarella cheese, ¼ cup roasted red peppers, 1 tsp. olive oil, ½ tsp. hot-pepper flakes, ¼ cup chopped sweet green peppers, ¼ cup chopped onions

〗 Spinach salad: ½ cup cooked white beans, 1 cup chopped spinach, and ½ carrot, chopped with 2 tsp. olive oil and 2 tbs. balsamic vinegar

〗 ½ cup seedless red grapes

Dinner

〗 3 oz. lean pork chops

〗 Potato sauté: 1 potato sliced, ¼ cup chopped shiitake mushrooms, ¼ cup chopped onions, 1 tbs. parsley, and 1 clove fresh garlic, minced, sautéed in ½ cup chicken stock

〗 Ratatouille: ¼ cup tomato sauce, ½ cup eggplant cubed, ¼ tomato chopped, ½ cup zucchini, ¼ cup chopped celery, served over ½ cup cooked orzo

〗 1 poached peach, sliced, with nutmeg and cinnamon

Snacks

〗 2 slices toasted cinnamon raisin bread

〗 2 fig bars

**Daily totals: 1,980 calories, 45 g fat (20 percent of calories),
13 g saturated fat (6 percent of calories), 116 mg choles-**

terol, 36 g dietary fiber, 9 g soluble fiber, 2,399 mg sodium, 936 mg calcium, 301 g carbohydrate (60 percent of calories), 100 g protein (20 percent of calories).

Day 6

Menu Tips

This menu has an omelette for dinner made from one egg and an egg substitute. The lunch can be eaten in a Chinese restaurant or purchased as a low-fat frozen entrée. Always check the sodium content. Most crackers or melba toast contain trans fat or hydrogenated fats, so read the ingredients on labels or else omit crackers from your diet. Carrots and apples are included for their soluble fiber. Eat them raw and cooked.

Breakfast

> ¾ cup orange juice or 1 orange
> 1 cup ready-to-eat oat cereal with ½ cup skim milk
> 1 banana

Lunch

> Egg drop or won ton soup: 1 cup hot, low-fat chicken broth with 2 tbs. egg substitute or wontons
> Chicken teriyaki with steamed vegetables or Buddha's delight (tofu with steamed vegetables)
> 1 cup steamed brown rice with chives
> ½ cup fresh or canned chunked pineapple, in juice

Dinner

> Omelette: ⅓ cup chopped mushrooms and ⅓ cup chopped onions, sautéed in 2 tsp. olive oil and folded into ¼ cup beaten egg substitute and 1 whole beaten egg

> 2 slices toasted whole-wheat bread with 2 tsp. diet mar-
> garine and 2 tbs. strawberry spread

> 1 apple, sliced, with 1 tbs. natural peanut butter

Snacks

> 1 slice multigrain bread

> 1 oz. low-fat Swiss cheese

> 1 pear

> ½ cup nonfat frozen chocolate yogurt

> Daily totals: 1,897 calories, 39 g fat (18 percent of calories),
> 8 g saturated fat (4 percent of calories), 268 mg choles-
> terol, 35 g dietary fiber, 8 g soluble fiber, 1,760 mg sodium,
> 921 mg calcium, 322 g carbohydrates (65 percent of calo-
> ries), 85 g protein (17 percent of calories).

Day 7

Menu Tips

Whole-grain cereal is the best choice. If you use a ready-to-eat variety, consider sprinkling some oat bran on top for the extra soluble fiber.

The goal per week is to have 7 ounces of high—omega-3 fatty acid fish, so the second serving of fish for this week is the tuna.

Breakfast

> 1 cup ready-to-eat frosted miniwheat or bran cereal with ½
> cup skim milk

> 2 slices toasted whole-wheat bread with 2 tsp. diet mar-
> garine

> 1 banana

Lunch

) ½ grapefruit

) Pasta salad: 1 cup cooked pasta, 3 oz. water-packed tuna, 1
oz. cubed low-fat cheddar cheese, ½ cup snow peas, ½ cup
frozen or canned plain artichoke hearts, and 2 chopped scallions, dressed with 1 tbs. low-fat mayonnaise, 1 tbs. vinegar,
fresh basil, and parsley

) 1 slice pumpernickel bread with 2 tsp. diet margarine

Dinner

) Chicken kabobs: 2 oz. cooked, cubed chicken breast with ¼
pepper, chunked, ½ tomato, chunked, 5 mushrooms, and ⅓
onion, chunked; marinated in 2 tsp. olive oil, 2 tsp. lemon
juice, 2 tsp. tamari soy sauce, 1 tbs. chopped parsley, 1
clove fresh garlic, minced, ¼ chili pepper, minced, and ¼
tsp. red-pepper flakes.

) 1 cup cooked whole-wheat couscous tossed with thyme or
parsley

) 1 low-fat ice cream sandwich

Snacks

) 1 cup grapes

) 1 oat bran and raisin muffin (2 oz.)

) 1 cup skim milk

> Daily totals: 1,904 calories, 49 g fat (22 percent of calories),
> 13 g saturated fat (6 percent of calories), 129 mg choles-
> terol, 38 g dietary fiber, 6 g soluble fiber, 2,084 mg sodium,
> 1,017 mg calcium, 297 g carbohydrates (59 percent of calo-
> ries), 93 g protein (19 percent of calories).

11

Drugs and Supplements

After a blood test, your doctor or other health professional will report your cholesterol levels. Get your own printed copy of the lab results and go over them with the doctor.

Depending on your scores and your risk factors, the doctor will have recommendations (see Chapter 4). If you have a high reading for total cholesterol and LDL, the doctor may recommend dietary changes, weight loss, exercise, or finally medication.

If you have one of the risk factors described earlier plus a family history of heart disease or high cholesterol, it would be important to lower both your total cholesterol and your LDL. After determining your chances of developing heart disease from the test in Chapter 5, you can decide what your goal will be.

Make a Commitment to Health

First, try to lower your cholesterol with diet and exercise, without medication. Ask your doctor how long you have to try this before the doctor would prescribe medication. The doctor may give you from four to six months to try to reduce your cholesterol by making better food choices, increasing the amount of exercise you get, stopping smoking, and/or losing weight. If after six months you see no change in cholesterol levels, the doctor will probably prescribe medication to achieve the necessary results.

If you already have heart disease or diabetes and your LDL (Low Down Lousy) cholesterol is above 100, changing your diet and exercising may not be enough. But you may be able to reduce your cholesterol by these means alone. Many people have. It does take a lot of commitment, and being willing to put health first, to see the importance of these life-saving changes, and then actually to carry them out. Lowering the fat content of your diet and your LDL level *can* shrink blockages in the arteries.

National Heart Lung and Blood Institute Drug Therapy Guidelines

Category I, Highest Risk

➤ You have heart disease, diabetes, or other risk factors.

➤ If your LDL is 100 or above, the TLC (Therapeutic Lifestyle Changes) diet will be recommended, possibly with drug therapy.

➤ If your LDL is 130 or higher, you will need to start drug therapy at the same time as the TLC diet.

Category II, Next-Highest Risk

➤ You have two or more risk factors for developing heart disease or having a heart attack.

➤ If your LDL is 130 mg/dL, you will need to begin the TLC diet.

➤ If your LDL is 130 mg/dL or higher after three months on the diet, you may need drug therapy and the TLC diet.

Category III, Moderate Risk

➤ You have two or more risk factors for heart disease and/or heart attack.

➤ If your LDL higher than 130, the TLC diet is recommended.

➤ If, after three months on the diet, your LDL cholesterol level is 160 mg/dL or higher, drug therapy may also be recommended to bring it down.

Category IV, Low-to-Moderate Risk

➤ You have one or no risk factor for heart disease and/or heart attack.

➤ If your LDL is 160 mg/dL or above, the TLC diet will be recommended.

➤ After three months of the diet alone, if your LDL level is still 160 mg/dL or higher, drug therapy may be recommended with the TLC diet, especially if your LDL cholesterol level is higher than 190 mg/dL.

Treatment With Drugs

The following sections describe the many drugs that are prescribed for cholesterol reduction. Before taking these or any other medications, be sure you have informed your health care professional about other conditions you have and medicines you are taking, including birth-control pills (statins, for example, can raise blood levels of birth-control hormones) and over-the-counter medications, vitamins, and nutritional supplements.

High-Fiber Supplements

The doctor may start you out on a high-fiber supplement such as psyllium or bran to try to lower your cholesterol. Two of the commercially branded laxatives that are basically high-fiber psyllium are Metamucil and Fiberall. As they pass through the system, they form a bulky mass that gathers cholesterol, which then passes out of the body along with the mass.

Citrucel, another bulk-forming laxative, contains methylcellulose, a high-fiber substance that prevents constipation and also moves fats and cholesterol out of the body.

Bile Acid Resins

The two main bile acid resins prescribed in the United States are Questran® and Colestid® (colestipol). They typically lower cholesterol by 10 to 20 percent. Questran (Bristol-Myers Squibb) is a cholestyramine resin. It belongs to a class of drugs called *bile acids sequestrants*, because they bind to bile acids in the digestive tract and carry them out of the body with the stool. Bile acids are made from cholesterol, and usually they are taken back into the bloodstream and recycled by the liver. When you take a bile acid sequestrant and the bile acids are removed from the body, the liver has to take cholesterol out of the blood to build new bile acids, and your blood cholesterol levels go down. Questran may also interfere with normal fat digestion and absorption.

Questran comes in powdered form. The powder is added to yogurt, pudding, applesauce, or orange juice, never taken as a dry powder. A bile acid resin may be prescribed in combination with another drug if you have high triglycerides or a history of severe constipation, because the bile acid resins tend to cause constipation.

One of the side effects of bile acid sequestrants is that they may delay or reduce the absorption of some oral medications and vitamins, for example, vitamins A, D, and K. For this reason, the resins and other medications should not be taken together. Other medications should be taken with different meals or different times of the day, at least one hour before, or four to six hours after taking a bile acid resin. Talk to a health care professional about the timing of this and any other medications you are taking.

If you are pregnant, your obstetrician may prescribe a special vitamin supplement. Always learn about possible side effects of medications and supplements, both prescription and nonprescription, and report any side effects to your doctor.

Welchol (colesevelam), another bile acid resin and cholesterol-lowering compound, is used along with diet and exercise. This medicine may take several weeks to begin showing an effect. Welchol has some side effects related to the stomach as well as muscle aches and weakness and is designed to be taken at lower doses than other bile acid resins. Welchol may be prescribed either alone or in combination with a statin.

Fibrates

These drugs reduce triglycerides by 20 to 50 percent and raise HDL cholesterol 10 to 15 percent. They are usually taken along with other cholesterol modification drug therapy. Fibrates include fenofibrate (Tricor) and gemfibrozil (Lopid).

Lopid is usually taken 30 minutes before breakfast and dinner. Side effects are rare, with nausea, gas, dizziness, stomach pain, and headache the most common. Fibrates may also increase the risk of cholesterol gallstones and can boost the effects of blood thinners.

Niacin

Another supplement the doctor may recommend is niacin (vitamin B_3). Only the nicotinic acid form of niacin taken in prescription doses will lower cholesterol: taking high doses on your own is not recommended. Always take niacin with your doctor's knowledge or advice.

The usual amount of niacin needed is 19 mg daily up to age 50 for men and 15 mg daily for men over 50. For women, it is 15 mg daily up until age 50, and then 13 mg daily.

Nicotinic acid has positive effects on cholesterol: it lowers LDL cholesterol by 10 to 20 percent and triglyceride levels by 20 to 50 percent, while lifting HDL cholesterol levels 15 to 35 percent.

High doses may cause skin flushing, rashes, stomach irritation, or liver damage. Nicotinic acid widens blood vessels, making flushing and hot flashes frequent side effects. You will probably develop a tolerance for the flushing or be able to lower its intensity by taking the drug with meals or using aspirin or a similar medication. Nicotinic acid can also intensify the effect of high blood pressure medication and produce various gastrointestinal problems—nausea, gas, vomiting, diarrhea, and activation of peptic ulcers. Serious side effects include gout and high blood sugar levels, with the risk increasing with an increase in the dose of the drug. There are also timed-release products that may not cause some of these side effects.

If you have diabetes, you will probably not be prescribed this drug, because it can raise blood sugar levels. Make sure your health care professional knows that you have diabetes if nicotinic acid is prescribed.

Niacin is found naturally in foods high in protein such as fish, poultry, legumes, and peanut butter and is also one of the vitamins that is used to enrich grain products.

Hormone Replacement Therapy?

The National Institute of Health and the National Cholesterol Education Program do *not* recommend using hormone replacement therapy as an alternative to cholesterol-lowering drugs.

The Statins

If the cholesterol-lowering methods you have tried do not budge your cholesterol or at least not enough, you may need finally to take a statin.

Statins were introduced in 1987, and now about 12 million Americans take some form of statin. Statins are highly effective cholesterol-lowering drugs that provide the added benefits of increasing HDL cholesterol somewhat and reducing triglyceride levels.

Statins work by inhibiting an enzyme called HMG-CoA reductase, which controls the rate at which the liver produces cholesterol. They also boost the liver's ability to remove LDL cholesterol from the blood. According to a heart disease researcher, they can prevent the need for bypass operations. In a group of patients who underwent stent implantation, those who had been receiving statin therapy had a 50 percent lower chance of experiencing a major cardiac event.

The statins are listed in the table below. Baycol is a statin that was voluntarily removed from the world market on August 8, 2001, by its manufacturer—Bayer A.G.—because of reports of a sometimes fatal severe muscle reaction.

Statin Types

Medication*	Statin Type	Manufacturer
Lescol (1993)	fluvastatin	Novartis/Sandoz
Lipitor (1996)	atorvastatin	Warner-Lambert
Mevacor (1987)	lovastatin	Merck and Co.
Pravachol (1991)	pravastatin	Bristol-Myers Squibb
Zocor (1991)	simvastatin	Merck and Co.

*Date approved by the Food and Drug Administration

When deciding whether or not to prescribe a statin for you, your doctor will probably not look only at your total cholesterol levels. The doctor will scrutinize your LDL and HDL levels as well. Dr. Norman Sarachek, a recently retired cardiologist, said that when deciding on therapy for his patients, "The HDL should be over 40 and the LDL should be less than 100." If the numbers are not this good (an HDL below 40 or an LDL above 100) and the person has a strong family history of heart disease, he prescribed Lipitor. "Diet will decrease cholesterol 15-20 percent, but statins will lower cholesterol 45 percent," was his opinion.

Dr. Sarachek says there are benefits to statins, over and

above lowering cholesterol. He himself takes a statin because he is interested in the ability of statins to reduce the incidence of stroke and heart attack. Although the cost is high, Dr. Sarachek believes the statins are worth taking.

Dr. Sarachek said he has seen few side effects with statins, maybe one in every 100 patients. He stopped the statin immediately when there were any side effects. The most common one is muscle aches. Liver enzymes should be checked periodically in anyone taking a statin.

The usual statin dose is taken with the evening meal, since the liver makes cholesterol mainly at night. It takes about four to six weeks on the statin to achieve the full effect. After six to eight weeks, your health care professional will check your LDL cholesterol and perhaps adjust your medication.

Statin Side Effects

Few people prescribed statins suffer serious side effects. The most common unwanted effects are upset stomach, gas, diarrhea, constipation, and abdominal pain or cramps. Some of the other side effects that can occur are rash, nausea, dizziness, headache, heartburn, blurred vision, or taste changes. The effects are usually mild to moderate in severity and fade as your body adjusts to the drug. However, if you experience brown urine or muscle soreness, pain or weakness, contact your health care professional immediately. Liver inflammation is a serious side effect, so a blood test to check liver enzyme levels should be done before taking statins, after six weeks on the drug, and then again after twelve weeks.

One other problem with these statins is their high price: the monthly cost can vary from $83 to $133.

Statins and Grapefruit Juice?

Statins should not be taken with grapefruit juice because there is a compound in the juice that prevents the drug from being absorbed and therefore used properly. If you enjoy grapefruit juice, take it at another time of the day, or at least two hours before or after taking the drug. You don't have to stop drinking it completely.

Statins and Alcohol?

Large amounts of alcoholic beverages, more than just a glass of wine a night, could increase the risk of liver damage, which is one of the side effects of the statins. The doctor will ask you to take a blood test regularly to make sure your liver is functioning properly.

Statins and Vitamin E?

Vitamin E is widely used to reduce the risk of heart disease because it is a powerful antioxidant. A recent study found that when vitamin E is taken along with a statin or niacin, the statin or niacin may not do its work properly. If you are taking a vitamin E supplement in addition to a statin, stop taking it.

If a Drug Is Prescribed, Take It

If your doctor prescribes a drug, make sure you take it as prescribed. It won't help if you get a prescription filled and then take it occasionally. These prescriptions are carefully worked out according to the results of studies, and if the doctor prescribes one pill at dinner, that is what you should take. Putting the pills on the table or in a little pill box for travel may help remind you to take a pill.

Other Cholesterol-Lowering Ideas

LDL Apheresis

LDL apheresis is a procedure that cleanses the blood of cholesterol. This procedure takes several hours while you are attached to equipment that removes the blood from the body, chemically cleanses it, and returns it to the body. The treatment must be repeated, usually every two to three weeks, and is time consuming and expensive.

Coenzyme Q_{10}

Some studies have shown that the statins interfere not only with the enzyme that is needed to produce cholesterol, but also with the body's production of coenzyme Q_{10} (CoQ_{10}). CoQ_{10} helps turn food into energy. It is produced in the body and is present in foods such as meat, fish, and soy oil.

Low levels of CoQ_{10} may depress heart function, and CoQ_{10} is used in some countries to treat heart failure. It is also used to enhance the effects of conventional drugs. Studies that examined the effects of statin drugs on the body's CoQ_{10} levels have found that people taking statin drugs have lower levels of CoQ_{10} in the blood.

Thus if you are taking a high dose of a statin, you may be decreasing the CoQ_{10} content of your blood, and supplemental CoQ_{10} may be in order. Talk to your physician about adding CoQ_{10} supplements, especially if you already have a problem with heart function. CoQ_{10} is fat-soluble and is better absorbed when taken in oil-based softgel form rather than in dry form such as tablets and capsules.

Combination Drug Therapy

If you haven't achieved your target LDL cholesterol level after six weeks on a single medication, your physician may recommend adding a second one or increasing the dosage. Various combinations have been shown to be effective and safe. Lower doses of each individual drug can reduce the risk of side effects.

Exercise, avoiding smoking, losing weight, and diet changes are still important along with the medication.

An HDL-Raising Idea

Studies are being performed on a new class of drugs that will raise the HDL cholesterol. At this writing, one successful test in the Netherlands resulted in raising the good cholesterol, the HDL, about 34 percent, with minor side effects of diarrhea or nausea. More studies will be necessary. Although the drug raises the HDL, it has not been shown to lower the risk of heart disease at this time.

APPENDIX

Where The Cholesterol and Fats Are Found

The following table shows the number of calories, total fat, saturated fat, trans fat, cholesterol, omega-3, and omega-6 fatty acid content of selected foods in several categories. A zero means there is no amount or no significant amount of that nutrient. A dash means that the amount is not available.

Food	Cal	Fat	Sat Fat	Trans Fat	Chol.	Omega-3	Omega-6
Meats							
Beef Ground, Lean 3 oz.	144	8	3	—	31	—	—
Beef, sirloin steak 3 oz. prime	213	16	7	.93	50	.16	.40
Ham, cured, roasted, 3 oz.	155	11	4	0	40	.11	1.04
Ham Sandwich (on white bread)	373	15	3	.57	49	.34	5.70
Hot dog, beef	180	16	7	.60	35	.15	.63
Hot dog, turkey	102	8	3	.08	48	.16	2.09
Pork chop, fried, 3 oz.	218	18	7	0	54	.10	1.81
Pork sausage, 2 oz.	183	15	5	.06	44	.25	1.61
Pork spareribs, 3 oz.	338	26	9	0	103	.09	2.23

Food	Cal	Fat	Sat Fat	Trans Fat	Chol.	Omega-3	Omega-6
Fish							
Sardines, in soy oil, 3 oz	177	10	1.3	0	120.8	1.26	3.01
Sardines, Skinless, boneless, 3 oz	185	11	2	0	70	1.95	0.22
Atlantic salmon, 3 oz.	121	5	0.8	0	47	1.5	0.4
Sockeye salmon, 3 oz.	130	6	1.4	0	37	1.1	0.4
Tuna light, Canned, in water, 3 oz.	99	.7	.2	0	26	0.2	0.04
Tuna, baked yellowfin, 3 oz.	118	1	.3	0	49	0.3	0.04
Haddock, 3 oz., steamed	94.4	.78	0.14	0	62	.20	0.03
Shrimp, steamed, 3 oz.	84	.9	0.18	0	166	0.4	0.06
Bluefish, 3 oz.	135	4.6	1.0	0	65	.84	.07
Poultry							
Chicken breast, skinless, boneless, 3 oz.	168	6.22	1.86	—	71	0.09	1.26
Chicken thigh, boneless, skinless, 3 oz.	178	9.25	2.58	—	81	0.14	1.9
Turkey, breast, skinless, boneless, 3 oz.	160	6.3	1.79	—	63	0.09	1.37
Turkey, dark, skinless, boneless, 3 oz.	106	3.7	1.25	0.12	59	0.06	1.04
Buffalo chicken wings, 6 pieces	295	21	6	—	78	0.38	4.77
Dairy							
Cheddar cheese ½ cup	266	22	14	0.6	69	0.24	0.38
Cheddar cheese, low-fat, ½ cup	114	4.62	2.87	—	13.86	0.04	0.10
Velveeta, 1 oz.	102	7.09	4.73	—	23.6	—	—
Velveeta, low-fat, 1 oz.	51	2	1.25	.06	9.92	0.02	0.04
Milk, whole, 1 cup	150	8.15	5.1	.22	33.18	.12	0.18

Food	Cal	Fat	Sat Fat	Trans Fat	Chol	Omega-3	Omega-6
Milk, 2-percent, 1 cup	121	4.68	2.93	0.13	18.3	0.07	0.10
Milk, 1-percent, 1 cup	102	2.59	1.61	0.07	9.76	0.04	0.06
Milk, 1 cup, skim	86	0.44	0.29	0.01	4.41	0	0.01
Ice cream, vanilla, ½ cup	133	7.3	4.5	0.2	29	0.11	0.17
Ice cream, Ben & Jerry's, ½ cup, Island Paradise	240	12	7	—	55	—	—
Ice cream. Haagen-Dazs, ½ cup, vanilla	270	18	11	—	120	—	—
Yogurt, frozen, soft-serve, chocolate, ½ cup	115	4.3	2.6	0	3.6	0.05	0.10
Yogurt, low-fat, plain, 1 cup	155	3.8	2.45	0.08	14.95	0.03	0.08

Fats and Dressings

Food	Cal	Fat	Sat Fat	Trans Fat	Chol	Omega-3	Omega-6
Butter, 1 tbs.	102	11.5	7.18	0	31	0.17	0.26
Margarine, 1 tbs., 60 percent oil/40 percent butter	101.4	11.35	4.04	1.56	12.5	0.10	2.16
Promise, 1 tbs., tub	101.7	11.42	1.82	—	0	0.06	6.76
Blue cheese salad dressing, 2 tbs.	154	16	3	—	5.2	1.13	7.2
Blue cheese Lo-cal salad dressing, 2 tbs.	30	2.2	0.79	—	0.31	0.09	0.65
Blue cheese Fat-free salad dressing, 2 tbs.	50	0	0	0	0	0	0

Vegetables, Beans, Soy

Food	Cal	Fat	Sat Fat	Trans Fat	Chol	Omega-3	Omega-6
Garlic , 1 clove	5	0.01	0	0	0	00	0.01
Carrot, 1	30.96	0.14	0.02	0	0	0.01	0.05
Tofu, ½ cup	94	5.93	0.87	0	0	0.40	2.96
Green soybeans raw, ½ cup	188	8.7	1.01	0	0	0.48	3.61
Soybeans, dry roasted, ¼ cup	194	9.29	1.37	0	0	0.62	4.64

Food	Cal	Fat	Sat Fat	Trans Fat	Chol.	Omega-3	Omega-6
Soybeans, black, canned, ½ c	90	1.5	—	—	0	—	—
Sweet potato baked and peeled	117.4	0.13	0.03	0	0	0.01	0.05
Watercress, ¼ cup chopped	1	0.01	0	0	0	0	0
Broccoli, ½ cup	12	0.15	0.02	0	0	.06	.02
Spinach, ½ cup chopped	3.3	.05	.01	0	0	.02	0

Grains

Food	Cal	Fat	Sat Fat	Trans Fat	Chol.	Omega-3	Omega-6
Barley, whole, cooked, ½ cup	97	.35	0.07	—	0	.02	.15
Oatmeal, cooked, ½ cup	73	1.1	0.2	—	0	.02	0.42
Brown rice long, cooked, ½ cup	108	0.88	0.18	—	0	.01	.30
Bulgur, cooked, ½ cup	76	0.22	0.04	—	0	0	.09

Nuts

Food	Cal	Fat	Sat Fat	Trans Fat	Chol.	Omega-3	Omega-6
English walnuts, chopped, ¼ cup	193	18.6	1.79	0	0	2.04	9.54
Almonds, whole, ¼ cup	207	19.63	1.38	0	0	0	3.31
Pistachio nuts, ¼ cup	184.64	15.49	2.01	0	0	0.08	2.25
Peanuts, raw, ¼ cup	206.95	17.96	3.06	0	0	0	5.69
Brazilnuts, 4	123.98	12.51	3.06	0	0	.01	4.50
Filberts/hazelnuts, Chopped, ¼ cup	181.7	18.0	1.33	0	0	0.04	1.68
Cashews, dry roasted, unsalted, ¼ c	196.6	15.89	3.19	0	0	0.06	2.62
Peanut butter smooth, 2 tbs.	189.76	16.32	3.58	—	0	0.02	4.38
Peanut butter, chunky, 2 tbs.	188.48	15.97	3.07	—	0	0.02	4.51

Food	Cal	Fat	Sat Fat	Trans Fat	Chol	Omega-3	Omega-6
Fruits							
Grapes, 1 cup	113	0.93	0.31	0	0	0.06	0.21
Fresh figs, three	111	0.45	0.09	0	0	0	0.22
Apple	81	0.50	0.08	0	0	0.02	0.12
Orange	61.57	0.16	0.02	0	0	0.01	0.02
Cakes, Desserts and Snacks							
Pudding, chocolate With milk, 2-percent, ½ cup	205.67	3.93	1.99	—	9.42	0.05	0.36
Doughnut, 1, cake type	198	10.8	1.8	2.28	17.4	0.26	3.57
Nachos, Taco Bell, 1 serving	320	18	4	—	5	—	—
Nachos, Taco Bell Big Beef Supreme, 1 serving	450	24	8	—	30	—	—
Pizza, Thick crust, 1/12 of 10-inch pie	489	10.45	4.66	0.37	26.1	0.16	1.45
Pizza Hut, Personal Pan Pizza Supreme	722	34	12.03	—	66	—	—
Triscuit cracker, 4	85.7	3.43	0.57	—	0	—	—
Peanut butter cookie, 1 homemade	95	4.76	0.89	—	6.2	.04	1.4
Hershey Mr. Goodbar, 1, 1.75 oz.	270	17.31	7.39	—	3.97	0	2.38
Hershey Reese's Peanut Butter Cup,1 mini	37.87	2.19	0.78	—	0.35	0	0.39
Hershey's cocoa powder, unsweetened, 1 tsp.	6.83	0.17	0.09	—	0	—	—

Above analyses from ESHA Research, Inc. Food Processor

REFERENCES

Introduction

Targeting the Facts, Our Quick Guide to Heart Disease, Stroke and Risks, American Heart Association 2002 Heart and Stroke Statistical Update, January 2, 2002, www.americanheart.org.

Chapter 1

Enig, Mary G. *Know Your Fats: The Complete Primer For Understanding the Nutrition of Fats, Oils and Cholesterol.* Silver Spring, MD: Bethesda Press, 2000.

Executive Summary of the National Cholesterol Education Program (NCEP) Expert Panel on Detection, Evaluation, and Treatment of High Blood Cholesterol in Adults (Adult Treatment Panel III) NIH Publication No. 01-3670, May 2001. www.nhlbi.nih.gov/guidelines/cholesterol.

Fallon, Sally and Mary G. Enig, Ph.D. "Inside Japan: Surprising Facts about Japanese Foodways." *Wise Traditions in Food, Farming, and the Healing Arts.* Publication of Weston A. Price Foundation, Washington, D.C., Fall 2001: 37.

Kenney, James, M.D. *Communicating Food For Health Newsletter.* Weston, FL. Copyright www.foodforhealth.com. April 2000.

Know Your Fats, scientific statement from the American Heart Association website, www.americanheart.org.

Lichtenstein, Ruch, D.Sc. "Transfatty Acids, Plasma Lipid Levels, and Risk of Developing Cardiovascular Disease." *Circulation* 95, (1997): 2588–2590.

Chapter 3

Duyff, Roberta Larson, M.S., R.D., CFCS. *The American Dietetic Association's Complete Food and Nutrition Guide.* Minneapolis, MN: Chronimed Publishing, 1996. pg 485.

"Good Fats, Bad Fats: New Insights into Diet and Health." *Harvard Men's Health Watch* 4, no. 10, (May 2000): 1–6.

Kenney, James, M.D. *Communicating Food For Health Newsletter.* Weston, FL. Copyright www.foodforhealth.com. April 2000.

Lehigh Valley Hospital Health Network. "Get on the Ball for Fitness." *Healthy You,* Allentown, PA. Jan/Feb 2002: 9.

Motsay, Stephen, M.D. "Triglycerides—The Other Bad Fat." *Healthy You,* Lehigh Valley Hospital and Health Network, Allentown, PA. Jan/Feb 2002: 5.

Tanne, David, et al: "Blood Lipids and First-Ever Ischemic Stroke/ Transient Ischemic Attack in the Bezafibrate Infarction Prevention (BIP) Registry: High Triglycerides Constitute an Independent Risk Factor." *Circulation: Journal of the American Heart Association* 104, (Dec. 11, 2001): 2892–2897.

Trubo, Richard, and Editors of *Prevention Magazine. Cholesterol Cures.* Emmaus, PA: Rodale Press, Inc., 1996.

Whitney, Eleanor Noss, Corinne Balog Cataldo, Sharon Redy Rolfes. *Understanding Nutrition,* 5th edition. Belmont, CA: West/Wadsworth, 1998.

Chapter 4

"On Whether to Have Your Homocysteine Level Measured." *Tufts University Health and Nutrition Letter* 16, No. 1, (March 1998): 3.

Schatz, I. J., Masakik, Yanok., et al. "Cholesterol and All-Cause Mortality in Elderly People from the Honolulu Heart Program: A Cohort Study." *Lancet* 358, (2001): 351–355

Chapter 6

McNamara, Donald J., Ph.D., ed. *Nutrition Close-Up*, Egg Nutrition Center 18, no. 4 (Winter 2001), www.enc-online.org.

Chapter 7

Stern, Lise. "Exchange Policy." *Cooking Light* 16, No. 1, (Jan/Feb 2002): 74.

Chapter 8

BMI chart from the National Heart, Lung and Blood Institute (NHLBI), "Clinical Guidelines on Overweight and Obesity." (June 1998). www.nhlbi.nit.gov/guidelines.

Chapter 9

"Dietary Approaches to Stop Hypertension." *Facts About the DASH Diet.* National Heart, Lung, and Blood Institute, NHLBI Health Information Center, PO Box 30105, Bethesda, MD 20824. www.nhlbi.nit.gov/health/public/heart/hbp/dash

Chapter 11

"Antioxidant Supplements Lose Promise as Disease Preventers." *Tufts University Health and Nutrition Letter* 20, No. 1:5.

Editors, Time-Life Books. *Time Life Medical Advisor: The Complete Guide To Alternative and Conventional Treatments.* Alexandria, VA, 1997.

ACKNOWLEDGMENTS

Thanks to Lois Young for her faithful reading of the manuscript and for giving invaluable practical suggestions, Nancy Schneider Burritt for her questions and support, and Martin Boksenbaum for being the devil's advocate. I appreciate my husband Sy, for his patience, and the rest of my family: Michael for editing the manuscript and giving freely of his excellent criticisms, and Lee and Scott for keeping me focused. Thanks to Scott Schneider and Martin Post for their stories; to Matthew Lore for his always excellent advice, especially suggesting I tell the cholesterol story as if I were talking to a friend; to Ellen Greene for her encouraging phone calls; to Gretchen Becker who whipped the manuscript into shape, and finally to JoAnne Steward, M.D., Norman Sarachek, M.D., and Dore Kottler, R.Ph.

Any nutrient data used in this book came from The Food Processor®Nutrition Analysis Software from ESHA Research, Salem, Oregon.

INDEX

About the Author

Anita Hirsch, M.S., R.D. has worked in the food and nutrition fields for thirty years—more than twenty of them spent developing and testing recipes for health books and magazines at Rodale Press. She has taught courses in food and cooking at the college level, and writes a "quick and healthy" column for several newspapers. Her previous books include *Drink to Your Health* (Marlowe & Company, 2000). She lives in Allentown, Pennsylvania.